MICROSCOPIC PROCEDURES
for Primary Care Providers

Shirley Lowe, MS, MT (ASCP)
Specialist, Department of Microbiology and Immunology
Assistant Clinical Professor,
Department of Community Health Systems
University of California at San Francisco
San Francisco, California

JoAnne M. Saxe, RN, C, ANP, MS
Adult Nurse Practitioner
Associate Clinical Professor
Department of Community Health Systems
School of Nursing
University of California at San Francisco
San Francisco, California

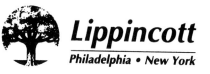

Lippincott
Philadelphia • New York

Acquisitions Editor: Lisa Stead
Sponsoring Editor: Claudia Vaughn
Senior Project Editor: Erika Kors
Senior Production Manager: Helen Ewan
Senior Production Coordinator: Nannette Winski
Assistant Art Director: Kathy Kelley-Luedtke

9 8 7 6 5 4 3 2 1

Library of Congress Cataloging-in-Publications Data
Lowe, Shirley
    Microscopic procedures for primary care providers/Shirley Lowe, JoAnne M. Saxe.
        p. cm.
    Includes bibliographical references and index.
    ISBN 0-7817-1432-X (alk. paper)
    1. Medical microscopy. 2. Primary care (Medicine) I. Saxe, JoAnne M. II. Title.
    [DNLM: 1. Laboratory Techniques and Procedures. 2. Microscopy—methods. 3. Primary Health Care—methods.   QY 25 L913m 1999]
RB43.L69 1999
6l6.07¹58—dc21
DNLM/DLC   98-22966
for Library of Congress   CIP

    Care has been taken to confirm the accuracy of the information presented and to describe generally accepted practices. However, the authors, editors, and publisher are not responsible for errors or omissions or for any consequences from application of the information in this book and make no warranty, express or implied, with respect to the contents of the publication.
    The authors, editors and publisher have exerted every effort to ensure that drug selection and dosage set forth in this text are in accordance with current recommendations and practice at the time of publication. However, in view of ongoing research, changes in government regulations, and the constant flow of information relating to drug therapy and drug reactions, the reader is urged to check the package insert for each drug for any change in indications and dosage and for added warnings and precautions. This is particularly important when the recommended agent is a new or infrequently employed drug.
    Some drugs and medical devices presented in this publication have Food and Drug Administration (FDA) clearance for limited use in restricted research settings. It is the responsibility of the health care provider to ascertain the FDA status of each drug or device planned for use in their clinical practice.

ACKNOWLEDGMENTS

We would like to thank the many students and faculty at the University of California at San Francisco, School of Nursing for their support, suggestions, and editorial comments during the evolution of this book. We would particularly like to thank Pat Jackson, RN, PNP, MS, Director of the Primary Nurse Practitioner Grant. We would also like to thank the Department of Microbiology at the University of California at San Francisco, for the use of its facilities, and IMS Photo for the use of its photomicroscope and excellent processing of the photomicrographs.

Many of the photographs in the book were taken by Shirley Lowe. A very few slides are old slides that are used for teaching at the University of California at San Francisco, where the photographer is unknown. We are grateful to Bayer Corporation for Figures 3-2, 3-6, 3-9, and 3-13; Meryl Haber for Figure 3-22; Sister Laurine Graff for the remaining urinalysis photos and Figure 7-10b; Raza Aly for Figures 7-2 and 7-4; Mike McGinnis for Figure 7-5; Thomas Garite and William N. Spellacy for Figure 7-7; and Judy Sakanari for Figure 7-10a.

Finally, and most importantly, we would like to acknowledge our families and friends, who provide an unending stream of love and support. Shirley would especially like to thank her husband, Dan Kipp, and her daughter, Katherine Clawson. She would also like to thank Carol Gross, Carlyn Halde, and Jill Cooper for their belief in her abilities and their constant encouragement. JoAnne would especially like to acknowledge her husband, Noel, and her daughters, Kelly, Jocelyn, and Lydia.

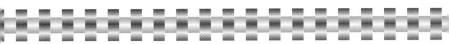

CONTENTS

Chapter 6

Collection and Handling of Endocervical and Urethral Specimens 149

Chapter 7

Miscellaneous Microscopic Examinations 167

Chapter 8

Diagnosis of Streptococcal Pharyngitis   193

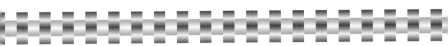

PREFACE

Clinicians often rely on common office-based laboratory tests, such as urinalyses, Gram stains, wet mounts, and rapid strepto-coccal antigen tests, to diagnose and manage health care conditions accurately. Successful selection and interpretation of these tests is dependent upon numerous variables:

- Proper collection and handling of specimens
- Appropriate use of diagnostic tools (eg, microscope, commercial testing kits, etc.)
- Accurate interpretation of test results with an appreciation of the sensitivity and specificity of the particular test
- Appreciation of time factors that influence availability and interpretation of test results, (Christenson & Overall, 1995)
- Knowledge of clinical decision making, including comprehension of important pathophysiologic, epidemiologic, psychosocial and clinical management concepts that help the clinician to determine which diagnostic tools are indicated given the patient's clinical presentation

This manual was written to address these variables and to provide the education and training needed to perform some common office laboratory tests. Studies have repeatedly shown that laboratory tests performed by individuals who have had no formal laboratory training are statistically less accurate and reliable (Grayson, 1984; Lunz, Castleberry, James, & Stahl, 1987) than tests performed by clinical laboratory scientists. A recent study done by the California Department of Health Services showed that physician office laboratories (POLs) in general had a significantly higher failure rate on proficiency test samples than non-POL laboratories. This study also showed that POLs that used RNs or other non–laboratory-trained individuals to perform laboratory testing had a higher failure rate than did POLs that employed licensed clinical laboratory scientists (California Department of Health Services, 1997). Studies have also shown that laboratory training programs can significantly improve testing accuracy (LaBeau, 1995; Murphy, Gessner, Macias, & Littlefield, 1983).

The authors have been teaching a laboratory methods class to advanced practice nursing students at the University of California, San Francisco for many years. This material has been determined to be an important component of their clinical education. Through the use of this learning manual, the students are able to provide accurate and reliable laboratory testing results.

There are many different laboratory tests that are performed by advanced practice nurses, physicians, and other healthcare practitioners. This manual makes no attempt to address all these laboratory tests. The testing procedures included in this manual have been chosen based on two factors. First, this manual is written primarily to instruct individuals on the use of a compound brightfield microscope and interpretation of specimens when examined microscopically. These tests have been categorized as "provider-performed microscopy tests (PPM)" by the "Clinical Laboratory Improvement Amendment of 1988—CLIA '88."

The second factor used to determine which tests to include in the manual is one of usage. Laboratory tests that are commonly performed in an office setting, such as dipstick testing of urine specimens and tests for the diagnosis of streptococcal pharyngitis, are also included.

Through the multi-experiential learning opportunities included in this manual, the reader should be able to achieve the following:

- Describe the components of a quality control program.
- Identify the features of a laboratory safety program.
- Manipulate a microscope.
- Perform a routine urinalysis (macroscopic, chemical, and microscopic).
- Prepare and interpret pH determinations, saline wet mounts, and potassium hydroxide mounts on vaginal secretions.
- Perform and interpret Gram stains.
- Describe the proper methods of collecting, handling, and processing of endocervical and urethral specimens.
- Perform and interpret a methylene blue stain for fecal leukocytes.

- Perform and interpret potassium hydroxide mounts on skin, hair, or nail scrapings.
- Perform and interpret a smear for the presence of pinworm ova.
- Perform and interpret pH determinations and the ferning test for detecting the presence of amniotic fluid.
- Perform a throat culture.
- Recognize and identify Group A beta-hemolytic streptococci from a throat culture.

To enhance learning and retention of this content, the manual uses well-supported learning strategies that encourage the reader to be actively engaged in the educational experience. First, each chapter has specific objectives that help the reader to identify promptly the expected learning outcomes. Second, through the use of pre- and post-tests for each chapter, the participant can readily measure his or her current knowledge base of the respective content area and immediate recall of the chapter's material. Also, retention of content along with the clinical application of the manual's material may be appreciated through the analyses of case studies, which are located in the appendix. All-in-all, this type of performance-based instruction provides the learner with a convenient, self-paced, immediate-feedback experience with an incorporation of both visual and kinesthetic learning approaches.

It is highly recommended that a practical laboratory session be taken along with this manual. Hands-on experience is an important component of skills learning.

REFERENCES

Christenson, J.C. & Overall, J.C. (1995). Proper use of the clinical microbiology lab. *Pediatrics in Review, 16*(2), 62–68.

California Department of Health Services. (1997). *Executive summary of physician office laboratory study.* Berkeley, CA: Laboratory Field Services.

Grayson, R.T. (1984). Effects of regulatory controls on the accuracy of clinical laboratory tests. *Journal of Medical Technology, 1*(8), 632–637.

LaBeau, K.M. (1995). Laboratory testing in previously unregulated laboratories. *Laboratory Medicine, 26*(1), 84–89.

Lunz, M.E., Castleberry, B.M., James, K., & Stahl, J. (1987). The impact of the quality of laboratory staff on the accuracy of laboratory results. *JAMA, 258*(3), 361–363.

Murphy, M.D., Gessner, D., Macias, G. & Littlefield, J. (1983). A clinical laboratory program to improve performance of resident physicians. *Clinical Laboratory, 2*(4), 321–327.

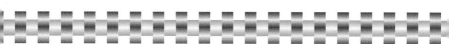

A USER'S GUIDE

This manual has been designed to provide a self-paced, skill-building learning opportunity that will prepare the participant to be able to perform a limited number of laboratory tests accurately at the completion of this instruction.

The reader who has the necessary knowledge and skills to meet each of the chapter's behavioral objectives may wish to proceed to the next chapter. For those users who need to acquire some or all of the knowledge and skills presented within the respective chapters, the authors suggest that they follow the sequence below:

1. Take the pre-test.
2. Identify the knowledge and skill deficits.
3. Read the chapter thoroughly, with special attention to the content that is new or needs reinforcement.
4. Take the posttest to assess mastery of content (the key is at the end of each chapter).

MICROSCOPIC PROCEDURES

for **Primary Care Providers**

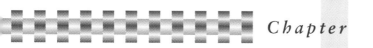

Quality Assurance and Laboratory Safety

Diagnosis and management of patient care is often based on laboratory test results. Therefore, it is important that laboratory tests be accurately done. One important factor in maintaining the accuracy of laboratory test results is adherence to a well-defined quality assurance (QA) program in the laboratory. To ensure reliable test results, it is important for clinicians to become familiar with the concepts of QA, and to develop and adhere to QA programs that fit the needs of the office laboratory.

Of equal importance is laboratory safety. Handling of potentially infectious material dictates that safety be a major concern in the office laboratory. All specimens tested must be considered potentially infectious and handled accordingly.

OBJECTIVES

Upon completion of this chapter, the reader will be able to:

1. Describe the federal and state regulations that govern the testing of human specimens in a clinical laboratory.
2. Summarize the regulations and significance of the Clinical Laboratory Improvement Amendment of 1988 (CLIA '88).
3. Describe the terms *waived tests, moderately complex tests, highly complex tests* and *provider performed microscopy tests.*
4. Describe the basic components of a quality assurance program.
5. Describe federal and state regulations that govern the safe handling of infectious material.

OBJECTIVES (Continued)

6. Discuss the concept of Standard Precautions as it applies to handling of patient specimens.

Please take the pretest. After completing the pretest, read the material in the chapter.

CHAPTER I PRETEST

1. What federal agency is responsible for the regulations that ensure a safe and healthful workplace?

2. Name the three categories of laboratory tests based on the complexity of the tests performed as established by CLIA '88.

Questions 3–5: Answer true or false.

3. Because proficiency testing is repeatedly done on a commercially available control sample, it is an internal check of the reliability of test results.

4. Provider performed microscopy (PPM) tests are moderately complex tests that may be performed by physicians, and other specified health care providers, on their own patients.

5. Food should be stored on a separate shelf in the laboratory refrigerator to lessen the chances of the food's becoming contaminated with reagents that may also be in the laboratory refrigerator.

The pretest answers will appear throughout the text of the chapter and before the posttest.

QUALITY ASSURANCE

All laboratories have an obligation to produce reliable test results. Large clinical laboratories and reference laboratories have had to follow a federally regulated set of guidelines to ensure accurate and reliable test results. Physician office laboratories (POLs) were exempted from such regulations. However, current legislation (**Clinical Laboratory Improvement Amendment of 1988 [CLIA '88]**) requires certification of POLs, including regulated quality assurance programs.

CLIA '88

In 1988, Congress passed the Clinical Laboratory Improvement Amendment (CLIA '88). This legislation set standards for all laboratory testing. Any facility that performs testing on human specimens for the purpose of diagnosis, assessment, or treatment is included in this legislation.

CLIA '88 regulations divide laboratory testing into the following three general categories based on the complexity of the testing procedure:

Waived tests: These are tests that "1) are cleared by FDA [Food and Drug Administration] for home use; 2) employ methodologies that are so simple and accurate as to render the likelihood of erroneous results negligible; or 3) pose no reasonable risk of harm to the patient if the test is performed incorrectly." (Federal Register, 1992, p. 7140)

In order to perform waived tests, a facility must acquire a certificate of waiver. With this certificate, the facility may perform only waived tests. Dipstick testing of urine specimens is the only waived test included in this manual. It appears because it is a commonly performed test and an integral part of a routine urinalysis.

Moderately complex tests and highly complex tests: These tests are significantly more difficult to perform than waived tests and, therefore, laboratories that perform them must acquire a certificate of compliance. The certificate of compliance requires adherence to regulations regarding standards for laboratory personnel, quality control and assurance, proficiency testing and on-site inspections to ensure compliance to the regulations.

▓ **Pretest question #2:** The three categories of laboratory tests are: waived, moderately complex, and highly complex.

The majority of laboratory tests fall into the moderately complex category. Certain very technically demanding procedures, such as western blot testing for human inmmunodeficiency virus (HIV) infection, are categorized as highly complex. The regulations for high and moderate complexity testing differ mainly in the standards for personnel and quality control.

Within the category of moderately complex tests is a subcategory called **Provider Performed Microscopy (PPM)**. The PPM category was established to allow a clinician to do specific microscopic analysis on his or her own patients without adhering to the costly and, some feel, burdensome regulations required of laboratories performing moderately complex tests. Many of the tests in this manual fall into the PPM category.

Tests in the PPM category are not included in the waived tests because they are not simple procedures. In order to be done properly, these tests require training and specific skills. "Personnel performing these tests must be proficient in the use of a microscope and must be able to detect and identify cellular elements in a specimen, both of which require substantial training, experience and specific knowledge to be accurately performed." (Federal Register, 1995, p. 20,036)

When first proposed, only physicians were allowed to perform tests within the PPM category. Because professional organizations representing other health care practitioners (nurse midwives, nurse practitioners, and physician assistants) pointed out that they also received the training necessary for carrying out such tests, the regulations were changed to allow these practitioners to perform the PPM tests as well.

▓ **Pretest question #4:** The following statement is true. Provider performed microscopy (PPM) tests are moderately complex tests that may be performed by a physician or other specified health care provider on his or her own patients.

This manual was developed to provide the instruction needed to perform competently the following PPM tests:

- Vaginal wet mounts
- KOH preparations
- Urine sediment examination
- Fecal leukocyte examination
- Pinworm analysis
- Fern test

Also included in this manual are several tests that do not fall into either the waived or the PPM category. They are the Gram stain and tests for the diagnosis of streptococcal pharyngitis. These tests are included in the manual because of the frequency with which they are done in POLs. The important thing to remember about these tests is that if they are going to be done in the office laboratory, then the laboratory must apply for and receive a certificate of compliance. As stated earlier, this requires adherence to regulations concerning standards for laboratory personnel, quality control, proficiency testing, and on-site inspections.

ELEMENTS OF A BASIC QUALITY ASSURANCE PROGRAM

A quality assurance (QA) program is a series of regularly followed procedures to prevent errors and ensure a certain degree of accuracy in test results. This can be done by monitoring every step in a test procedure from the collection of the specimen to the reporting of the result. QA involves all aspects and areas of laboratory testing: preanalytical, analytical, and postanalytical. In order to ensure reliable test results, the following elements must be routinely monitored and adequate records kept:

Procedure Manual: Every laboratory must have a procedure manual that describes all procedures performed in that laboratory. The procedure manual should be reviewed and updated yearly.

Maintenance of Equipment: There should be a continuous plan for maintenance of all equipment in the laboratory. A log of routine maintenance, malfunctions, and corrective actions should be kept on all equipment.

Specimen Collection and Handling: All specimens should be properly collected and labeled. Procedure manuals must include information about what types of specimens are acceptable for each test that will be done in the laboratory and how the specimens should be handled before testing.

Quality Control Program

According to CLIA '88, "The laboratory must establish and follow written quality control procedures for monitoring and evaluating the quality of the analytical testing process of each method to assure the accuracy and reliability of patient test results and reports." (Federal Register, 1992, p. 7163) An acceptable quality control program must include the following:

Control of reagents and materials: In order to ensure reliable results, the reagents, materials, and supplies must be monitored. They must be stored properly and never used after their expiration date.

Use of control specimens: Control specimens should be used whenever possible to determine the reliability of a test. A control is a specimen of known value that is similar in composition to the unknown specimen. For example, if you need a control for routine dipstick testing of urine specimens, then you should use a control that is similar in composition to urine. The control specimen must be handled and tested in the same manner in which the unknown specimens are handled.

Test results and reporting: The laboratory must maintain a record of all patient test results. Also, a procedure must be in place for reporting test results, in a timely manner, to the appropriate person. Confidentiality of all test results must be ensured.

Proficiency testing: Proficiency testing is an "external" check on the quality of testing being done in the laboratory. It involves receiving unknown samples from a licensed provider. These samples are tested in the same manner in which specimens are tested in the laboratory, and the results are sent to the provider. Proficiency testing programs are available from many professional societies. Waived tests and PPM tests do not require proficiency testing.

■ **Pretest question #3:** The following statement is false. Because proficiency testing is repeatedly done on a commercially available control sample, it is an internal check of the reliability of test results.

Education of Personnel

Many studies have shown that the competency of testing personnel is an important determinant of the accuracy of laboratory testing. (California Department of Health Services, 1997; Grayson, 1984; LaBeau, 1995; Lunz, Castleberry, James, & Stahl, 1987). CLIA '88 regulations require laboratories to "ensure that prior to testing patients' specimens, all personnel have the appropriate education and experience, receive the appropriate training for the type of complexity of the services offered, and have demonstrated that they can perform all testing operations reliably to provide and report accurate results." (Federal Register, 1992, p. 7173)

CLIA '88 regulations also require laboratories to have policies established for monitoring the competency of all personnel performing laboratory tests and, whenever necessary, to provide remedial training or continuing education to improve skills.

LABORATORY SAFETY

Standards for laboratory safety are regulated by federal, state, and local agencies. The regulations are designed to protect people working in the laboratory, other health-care personnel, patients, the environment and, thus, society as a whole.

The **Occupational Safety and Health Administration (OSHA)** regulates the workplace to ensure that personnel have a safe working environment. The OSHA standard mandates the use of **Standard Precautions** when working with patients or handling human specimens. Standard Precautions are a set of recommendations from the **Centers for Disease Control and Prevention** to protect health-care workers and others from acquiring work-related infections.

▨ **Pretest question #1:** The federal agency responsible for regulations that ensure a safe and healthy workplace is OSHA, the Occupational Safety and Health Administration.

Standard Precautions require that every direct contact with body fluids from every patient be considered potentially infectious. Thus, **all** contact with body fluids from **all** patients should be handled in the same manner. Copies of the regulations are available from CDC (CDC, 1988; 1994).

General Laboratory Safety Rules

- Smoking, eating, and drinking are prohibited in the laboratory.
- Food must not be stored in laboratory refrigerators, nor should food be kept in any other area of the laboratory except in "clean" areas designated for food storage.

Pretest question #5: The following statement is false. Food should be stored on a separate shelf in the lab refrigerator to lessen the chances of the food becoming contaminated with reagents that may also be in the laboratory refrigerator.

- Pipetting by mouth is prohibited. Special pipetting devices are commercially available and should *always* be used.
- Disposable gloves should be worn when handling patient specimens.
- A laboratory coat or other appropriate protective clothing should be worn. This coat should not be worn in other areas of the office.
- WASH HANDS OFTEN. Be sure to wash your hands every time you leave the laboratory. Handwashing is the single most effective way to prevent the transmission of most infectious microorganisms.
- Laboratory counters should be disinfected regularly.

Special Safety Equipment

Because of the nature of the laboratory, certain equipment must be available to ensure the safety of personnel:

- Fire extinguisher
- Fire blanket
- Eyewash

Disposal of Infectious Material

The proper techniques for the disposal of contaminated waste are governed by OSHA, the **Environmental Protection Agency (EPA),** and state and local regulations.

All potentially infectious material must be decontaminated before disposal. This is most effectively done by autoclaving or incineration. It is impractical for most office settings to have an autoclave large enough for disposal purposes. Therefore, it is recommended that all contaminated materials be placed in a special biohazard container lined with an autoclavable bag. Arrangements can then be made with a local hospital or reference laboratory to autoclave the filled biohazard bags.

All glass (pipettes, slides, tubes etc.) should be disposed of in puncture resistant boxes. When full, these boxes should be taped shut and autoclaved before disposal.

CHAPTER I PRETEST ANSWERS

1. The federal agency responsible for regulations that ensure a safe and healthy workplace is OSHA, the Occupational Safety and Health Administration.

2. The three categories of laboratory tests are: waived, moderately complex, and highly complex.

3. False. Proficiency testing is done on samples from an outside provider and thus is an "external" check of reliability. Proficiency testing samples should be treated just as any patient specimen and, therefore, should not be done repeatedly.

4. This is a true statement.

5. False. Food should never be stored in a laboratory refrigerator. A separate "clean" refrigerator should be available for food storage.

CHAPTER I POSTTEST

1. Describe the principle of Standard Precautions.

2. Categorize the following tests as waived, moderately complex, or highly complex. If moderately complex, also indicate whether it is in the PPM category.

   a. Dipstick urinalysis

   b. Microscopic urinalysis

   c. Gram stain

   d. Vaginal wet mount

Questions 3–7: Fill in the blank.

3. _____ is a continuing process that includes all areas of the laboratory (preanalytical, analytical, and postanalytical) to prevent errors and ensure accurate test results.

4. Two methods that can be used to decontaminate infectious material effectively are _____ and _____.

5. A _____ is a sample of known value that is similar in composition to unknown specimens and is used to indicate the reliability of a testing procedure.

6. _____ is the single most effective procedure that can be done to prevent the transmission of most infectious agents.

7. _____ are federal regulations that set standards for all laboratories that do testing on human specimens for diagnosis, treatment, or management. The standards are designed to ensure accurate laboratory test results and quality patient care.

CHAPTER 1 POSTTEST ANSWERS

1. Standard precautions are recommended safety procedures and policies used for handling **all** patient specimens. Infectivity of any patient's specimens is unknown and therefore all blood and body fluid specimens should be considered equally infectious and treated accordingly.

2. a. Dipstick urinalysis—Waived test
   b. Microscopic urinalysis—Moderately complex and PPM
   c. Gram stain—Moderately complex
   d. Vaginal wet mount—Moderately complex and PPM

Questions 3–6: Fill in the blank.

3. *Quality assurance* is a continuing process that includes all areas of the laboratory (preanalytical, analytical, and postanalytical) to prevent errors and ensure accurate test results.

4. Two methods that can be used to decontaminate infectious material effectively are *incineration* and *autoclaving*.

5. A *control sample* is a sample of known value that is similar in composition to unknown specimens and is used to indicate the reliability of a testing procedure.

6. *Handwashing* is the single most effective procedure that can be done to prevent the transmission of most infectious agents.

7. *Clinical Laboratory Improvement Amendment of 1988 (CLIA '88)* is a set of federal regulations that establishes standards for all laboratories that do testing on human specimens for diagnosis, treatment, or management. The standards are designed to ensure accurate laboratory test results and quality patient care.

REFERENCES

California Department of Health Services. (1997). *Executive summary of physician office laboratory study*. Berkeley, CA: Laboratory Field Services.

Centers for Disease Control (CDC). (1987). Recommendations for prevention of HIV transmission in health-care settings, 1987. *Morbidity and Mortality Weekly Report Supplement, 36*, 25–185.

Centers for Disease Control (CDC), (1992). Regulations for Implementing the Clinical Laboratory Improvement Amendments of 1988: A Summary, 1992. *Morbidity and Mortality Weekly Report. 41*(RR-2), 1–16.

Centers for Disease Control and Prevention (CDC). (1994). Draft guideline for isolation precautions in hospitals: Part II. Recommendations for isolation precautions in hospitals. *Federal Register*, (Nov. 7, 1994), 59, 55552–55570.

Clinical Laboratory Improvement Amendment of 1988, final rule. (1992). 42 CFR Part 405, et al. *Federal Register*, (Feb. 28 1992), 7,002–7,186.

Clinical Laboratory Improvement Amendment of 1988. (1995). 42 CFR Part 493. *Federal Register*, (Apr. 24 1995), 20,035–20,053.

Grayson, R. T. (1984). Effects of regulatory controls on the accuracy of clinical laboratory tests. *Journal of Medical Technology, 1*, 632–637.

LaBeau, K. M. (1995). Laboratory testing in previously unregulated laboratories. *Laboratory Medicine, 26*, 84–89.

Lunz, M. E., Castleberry, B. M., James, K., & Stahl, J. (1987). The impact of the quality of laboratory staff on the accuracy of laboratory results. *JAMA, 258*, 361–363.

Basic Microscopy

Most primary care clinicians use a compound brightfield microscope in their practices, yet few have been trained in the use of this precision instrument. This chapter will provide an introduction to the components, operating principles, and proper care of the microscope.

A compound microscope is one with multiple lens systems. Clinical microscopes have two lens systems that provide magnification: the objectives and the oculars.

The term "brightfield" refers to the type of illumination. In brightfield microscopy, cells or structures in the specimen appear dark against a bright background.

OBJECTIVES

Upon completion of this chapter, the reader will be able to:

1. Locate the following components on a compound, brightfield microscope: condenser, aperture diaphragm, stage, coarse and fine focus adjustment knobs, oculars, and objectives.
2. Describe the functions of the above-mentioned components.
3. Name and calculate the final magnification of the three objectives most often present on clinical microscopes.
4. Describe the proper techniques used to focus a microscope when studying unstained wet-mount specimens and stained specimens.
5. Discuss the proper care and maintenance of a microscope.
6. Identify and solve common problems encountered when using a microscope.

OBJECTIVES (Continued)

Please take the pretest. After completing the pretest, read the material in the chapter.

CHAPTER 2 PRETEST

1. Label the following parts of the microscope on the diagram below: condenser, objectives, stage, fine-adjustment knob (Fig. 2-1).

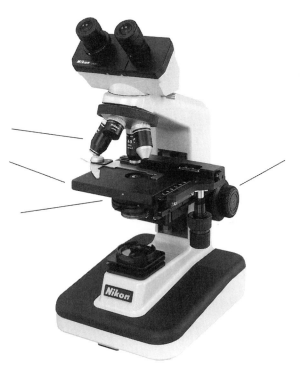

FIGURE 2-1
Pretest question #1.

Questions 2–4: Answer true or false.

2. In order to focus and use the microscope properly, people who wear eyeglasses should keep them on when looking through the microscope.

3. When using the oil-immersion lens, a drop of oil is placed on the top of the condenser, and the condenser is raised until the drop of oil hits the bottom of the slide.

4. When looking at wet-mount specimens, the condenser of the microscope should be raised to just below the slide and the aperture diaphragm should be mostly closed.

Question 5: Multiple choice. Select the one best answer.

5. When microscopically looking at urine sediment, cells are enumerated using the

    a. scanning objective.

    b. low-power objective.

    c. high-power objective.

    d. oil-immersion objective.

The pretest answers will appear throughout the text of the chapter and before the posttest.

DESCRIPTION OF THE MICROSCOPE

In order to use the microscope properly, it is necessary to understand its parts and their functions. Although all microscopes are not identical, there are so many similarities that the following descriptions and pictures can serve as a general guide.

The microscope can be divided into four basic component systems (Fig. 2-2).

- Support system
- Illumination system
- Magnification system
- Adjustment system

Support System

The support system is the skeleton of the microscope, the part that holds it all together. It is composed of the base, support arm, stage,

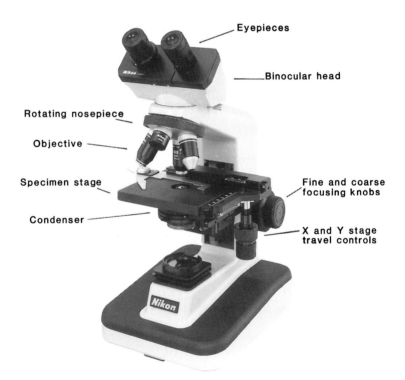

FIGURE 2-2
Compound brightfield microscope. (Photo courtesy of Nikon Inc., Instrument Division.)

and substage assembly. The base and support arm are fairly obvious. The stage and substage are described in this section (Fig. 2-3).

STAGE

The stage is the surface on which the microscope slide is placed. For clinical work a mechanical stage is preferred. This type of stage allows you to move the slide in a smooth and controlled manner. The stage movement is controlled by two knobs on the side of the microscope (Fig. 2-4). One knob moves the stage from left to right and one knob moves the stage up and down. Some older or less expensive microscopes may have a manual stage. With this type of stage, you hold the slide between your fingers and manually move the slide on the stage. It is very difficult to control the movement of the slide with this type of stage.

To position the slide in the slide holder, gently pull back the long arm of the slide holder, place the slide against the back of the holder and then slowly release the long arm.

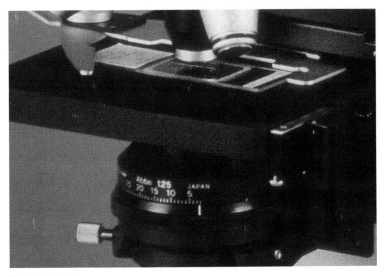

FIGURE 2-3
Stage and substage. (Photo courtesy of Nikon Inc., Instrument Division.)

SUBSTAGE

The substage assembly holds the condenser. The condenser can be raised or lowered using the condenser adjustment knob, usually located on the left side of the condenser (see Fig. 2-4).

Illumination System

The most common problem in office microscopy is incorrect adjustment of the illumination system. The illumination system consists of three components; the condenser, the aperture diaphragm, and a light source.

LIGHT SOURCE

The routine clinical microscope is called a brightfield microscope. The term brightfield refers to the type of illumination used. Modern brightfield microscopes use an incandescent, tungsten, or halogen bulb as a light source. The light intensity is con-

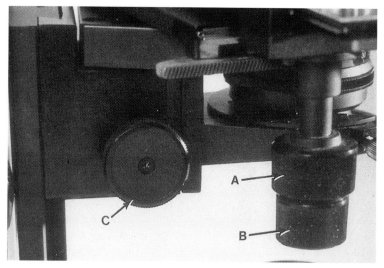

FIGURE 2-4
Stage (A and B) and Condenser (C) control knobs. Reprinted with permission from Smith, R.F. (1993). *Microscopy and photomicroscopy.* Boca Raton: CRC Press.

trolled by a rheostat, usually located on the base of the microscope. The light intensity should normally be set in the upper middle range.

CONDENSER AND APERTURE DIAPHRAGM

The light from the bulb passes through the condenser, which focuses the rays of light on the slide to be studied. The condenser must be adjusted correctly in order to focus the microscope properly. The position of the condenser is controlled by turning the control knob, usually located on the left side of the condenser (see Fig. 2-4). As a general rule, the condenser should be raised to a position just below the stage. Raise the condenser to its highest position (closest to the stage) and then lower the condenser slightly by turning the condenser adjustment knob about an eighth of a turn.

The angle of the light rays entering the condenser is regulated by the **aperture diaphragm** (also called the iris diaphragm) located on the condenser. The angle of the light entering the condenser affects the resolution and contrast of the specimen you are viewing.

IMPORTANT DEFINITIONS

Contrast.   Refers to the ability to detect differences in density. In unstained specimens, the identification of cells, structures within cells, and so on is often dependent upon subtle differences in density, (eg, the nucleus of a white blood cell is denser than its cytoplasm). The condenser and aperture diaphragm control the contrast.

Resolution.   Refers to the ability of the microscope to show detail, or the smallest distance between which two points can be separately identified. In other words, if there are two dots in the field and you have good resolution, you will see two dots (. .). If you have poor resolution, the two dots may appear as one blurred line (—). If there is too much light (aperture diaphragm opened too wide), there is little contrast between the image and the background, which results in poor resolution. By closing the aperture diaphragm, contrast between the object and the background can be increased and resolution is enhanced. Too much contrast (aperture diaphragm is closed too much) will decrease the resolution and lead to blurred images.

⫿⫿⫿⫿ Clinical Tip

- Generally, when studying **stained specimens**, the **condenser should be raised** and the **aperture diaphragm should be mostly opened.**
- When studying **unstained specimens**, such as wet preps or urine sediments, the **condenser should be raised** and the **aperture diaphragm should be mostly closed** to give optimum contrast.
- More detailed instructions about the use of the condenser can be found in the section "Use of the Microscope."

▪ **Pretest question #4:** The following statement is true. When looking at wet-mount specimens, the condenser of the microscope should be raised to just below the slide and the aperture diaphragm should be mostly closed.

Magnification System

A compound microscope has two separate lens systems that provide magnification, the ocular lenses (eyepiece) and the objective lenses. The total magnification is determined by multiplying the ocular magnification by the objective magnification.

OCULAR LENSES

The ocular lenses are the lenses that you look into. Most clinical microscopes are binocular, meaning they have two eyepieces. Magnification in the eyepiece lenses is usually $10\times$.

OBJECTIVE LENSES

There are three objective lenses on most clinical microscopes. The objectives are attached to a revolving nosepiece. To change from one objective to another you simply turn the nosepiece until the objective you want is directly over the slide and clicked into place (Fig. 2-5; Table 2-1).

Some microscopes have a fourth objective called a scanning objective. It provides $4\times$ magnification and is used to view large tissue sections. This objective is not used routinely by most health care providers for clinical laboratory tests.

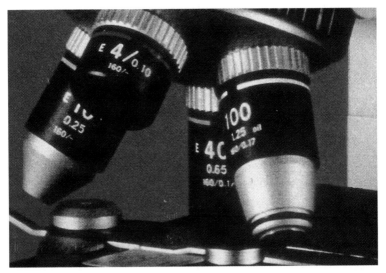

FIGURE 2-5
Nosepiece with objectives. (Photo courtesy of Nikon, Inc., Instrument Division.)

Low Power (10×)

This objective is used to focus the microscope and scan specimens to get a general idea of the type of specimen you have. For example, examination of a urine sediment with the low-power objective may show many epithelial cells. This indicates that the specimen has been contaminated with vaginal secretions and is not a

TABLE 2-1. Magnification of Microscope Objectives		
	Objective Magnification	Total Magnification
Low-power objective	10X	10 X 10 = 100
High-power objective	40X	40 X 10 = 400
Oil-immersion objective	100X	100 X 10 = 1000

good, clean-catch specimen. The low-power objective is also used to quantitate casts in urine sediments. A microscopic urine report may read, "1–3 hyaline casts per LPF (low-power field)." It is usually not possible to differentiate cells under low power. For that a high-power objective is needed.

HIGH POWER (40×)

This objective is used to differentiate cells and structures in "wet" specimens (ie, vaginal wet mounts and urine sediments). The high-power objective is used to quantitate cells, bacteria, yeast, and so forth in urine sediments and wet-mount preparations. (For example, 3–5 white blood cells per high-power field [HPF]. This objective is also called the high-dry objective.

■ **Pretest question #5:** The answer is c, high-power objective.

When microscopically looking at urine sediment, cells are enumerated using the high-power objective.

OIL IMMERSION (100×)

This is the objective used to look at stained specimens such as Gram stains. To use this objective, a drop of immersion oil must be placed on the top of the slide (the oil will provide a connection between the slide and the objective). Always use **immersion oil** and not mineral oil when using this objective. Also, this objective is the only one that is specially sealed so that the oil will not seep into the objective. Therefore, do not use the high-power (40×) objective when there is oil on the slide. If immersion oil gets on any of the other objectives, you should immediately wipe it off the objective with lens paper. Table 2-1 sumarizes the objective lenses.

■ **Pretest question #3:** The following statement is false. When using the oil-immersion lens, a drop of oil is placed on the top of the condenser, and the condenser is raised until the drop of oil hits the bottom of the slide.

Most microscopes are **parfocal**. This means that once the microscope is in focus using one objective, it should remain very close to being in focus when changed to a new objective. This is discussed in more detail in the section "Use of the Microscope."

Adjustment System

The adjustment or focusing system allows you to focus the microscope on the slide to be studied. The microscope is focused using two adjustment knobs located on the side of the microscope (see Fig. 2-2). The outermost knob is the coarse-adjustment knob. Turning this knob will grossly move the slide closer to or further from the objective. The innermost knob is the fine-adjustment knob. Turning this knob will result in very slight movements.

There are also adjustments that can be made to one of the ocular lenses of the microscope to accommodate differences in visual acuity of the two eyes of the microscopist. On most microscopes, one of the oculars will have a ribbed band around it (Fig. 2-6). This ocular can be separately focused on the slide to be studied. To focus this ocular, close the eye that looks into the ribbed ocular and focus the microscope using the procedure discussed on page 26. After the microscope is focused on the slide, open the eye that is looking through the ribbed eyepiece and close the other eye. Turn the ribbed band (not the whole eyepiece) until the slide is again in focus. Then open both eyes; the slide should be in sharp

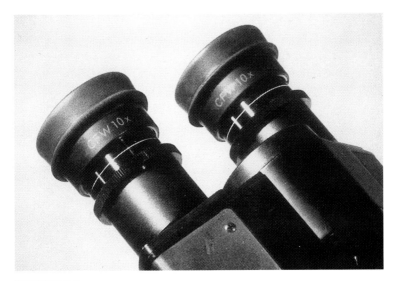

FIGURE 2-6
Oculars. Reprinted with permission from Smith, R.F. (1993). *Microscopy and photomicroscopy.* Boca Raton: CRC Press.

focus. It is not necessary to refocus the eyepiece each time you change the slide. However, if someone else uses the microscope, refocusing of the eyepiece may be necessary.

USE OF THE MICROSCOPE

Examining "Wet" Specimens (Vaginal Wet Mounts, Potassium Hydroxide [KOH] Mounts, and Urine Sediment)

1. Turn the microscope on and set the light intensity in the upper middle range.
2. Rotate the nosepiece so that the low-power (10×) objective is locked into position.
3. Raise the condenser on the microscope to its highest position and then lower it about an eighth of a turn. Close the aperture diaphragm.
4. Place the slide on the microscope stage and secure it between the fingers of the slide-holder assembly.
5. Before looking through the microscope, use the coarse-adjustment knob to move the stage upward so that the lens is about 1/4 inch from the slide.
6. Using both eyes, look through the microscope and turn the coarse-adjustment knob to increase the distance between the slide and the lens until something flashes into focus. (To avoid smashing the objective into the slide, always increase the distance between the slide and the objective while you are looking in the microscope.)
7. Use the fine-focus knob to sharpen the focus. If necessary, focus the ocular with the ribbed band to accommodate differences in the visual acuity of your two eyes (see section on adjustment system—pp. 25–26).
8. Use the low-power (10×) objective to scan the specimen. To look at different fields, move the slide by turning the knobs that control the slide-holder assembly. As you move from field to field, it will be necessary to keep focusing with the fine-focus knob. Continually turn the fine-focus knob back and forth to ensure that you are seeing the whole depth of field.
9. To use the high-dry (40×) objective, rotate the nosepiece until the lens clicks into position. Most microscopes are

parfocal, meaning that if a specimen is in focus under low power, it will be almost in focus when changed to a new objective. Only slight adjustment of the fine focus is generally required to bring the image into sharp focus.

When looking at wet specimens, you should not use the oil-immersion lens. As the magnification increases, so does the length of the objective. The oil-immersion lens is the longest of the objectives and it can break the coverslip, resulting in loss of the specimen or damage to the objective.

10. You may need to increase the light when increasing magnification. You can increase the light by opening the aperture diaphragm slightly until optimum contrast is achieved.

Examining Stained Slides

1. Turn the microscope on and set the light intensity in the upper middle range.
2. Rotate the nosepiece so that the low-power (10×) objective is locked into position.
3. Raise the condenser on the microscope to its highest position and then lower it about an eighth of a turn. Open the aperture diaphragm.
4. Place the slide on the microscope stage and secure it between the fingers of the slide-holder assembly.
5. Before looking through the microscope, use the coarse-adjustment knob to move the stage upward so that the lens is about 1/4 inch from the slide.
6. Using both eyes, look through the microscope and turn the coarse-adjustment knob to increase the distance between the slide and the lens until something flashes into focus. (To avoid smashing the objective into the slide, always increase the distance between the slide and the objective while you are looking in the microscope.)
7. Use the fine-focus knob to sharpen the focus. If necessary, focus the ocular with the ribbed band to accommodate differences in the visual acuity of both eyes (see section on adjustment system—pp. 25–26).
8. Use the low-power (10×) objective to scan the specimen. To look at different fields, move the slide by turning the knobs that control the slide-holder assembly.

9. Find an area of the slide that you want to examine more closely. Put a cell or structure (something to focus on) in the center of the field.

10. Place a small drop of immersion oil on the section of the slide that you will be examining with the oil-immersion lens. Turn the objective nosepiece to the 100X objective. **Do not drag the 40× objective through the drop of oil. If this happens, immediately clean the oil off the objective using lens paper.** Most microscopes are parfocal, meaning that if a specimen is in focus under low power, it will be almost in focus when changed to a new objective. Only slight adjustment of the fine focus is generally required to bring the image into sharp focus.

11. As you move from field to field, it will be necessary to keep focusing with the fine-focus knob. Continually turn the fine-focus knob back and forth to ensure that you are seeing the whole depth of field.

COMMON QUESTIONS AND PROBLEMS IN MICROSCOPY

Questions

Q: Should I wear my glasses when looking through a microscope?

A: If you are nearsighted or farsighted, you should take your glasses off when using the microscope. If you have an astigmatism, however, you may need to wear your glasses, because the microscope cannot adjust for astigmatism. Bifocals should not be worn when doing microscopy.

■ **Pretest question #2:** The following statement is false. In order to focus and use the microscope properly, people who wear eyeglasses should keep the eyeglasses on when looking in the microscope.

Q: Should I use both eyes when I look through the microscope?

A: Yes, you should look through the microscope with both eyes. Many people have difficulty using both eyes when looking through the microscope. Instead of seeing one large, round field, they see two separate, small round fields. There are several adjustments that can be made to bring the two fields together.

First, the eyepieces can be moved closer together or farther apart to adjust for differences in the distance between your eyes.

Also, when looking through the microscope, do not put your eyes directly against the eyepieces. Pull your head back a little from the microscope. Many times this will join the two fields.

Q: How bright should I set the light when using the microscope?

A: How high you set the intensity of the light source is generally based on personal preference. However, there are some general rules to follow. The light intensity should be high enough to illuminate the field adequately. The field should be bright, but not blinding. Generally, the higher the magnification, the more light you need. So as you increase magnification, you also need to increase your light intensity.

Problems

Problem: The microscope focuses with the low (10×) or high-dry (40×) power, but not with the oil-immersion lens.
Solution: First try adding another drop of oil. If this doesn't work, flip the slide over; it may be on the stage upside down.

Problem: All you can see is a white background with a patterned, gray speckling.
Solution: Lower the condenser just a little; the condenser is too close to the slide.

Problem: The image is not sharp.
Solution: If using the 40× (high-power) objective, clean it. There may be oil on the objective. If using the 100× (oil-immersion) objective, place a drop of oil on the slide. Oil is necessary to obtain a sharp focus with the 100× objective.

Problem: The field is obscured by concentric gray circles or black lines that do not move when you move the slide.
Solution: Clean the oculars with lens paper. Fingerprints and mascara from eyelashes often deposit on the eyepieces.

CARE OF THE MICROSCOPE

A microscope is a precision instrument and should be treated accordingly. It may appear to be indestructible, but in reality the slightest jar may damage its working parts and optical system. It is essential that the microscope be kept clean and in good working condition.

- Always carry the microscope in an upright position. Hold the arm of the microscope with one hand and support the base with the palm of the other hand.
- A clean microscope is a happy microscope and will provide you with years of service. The most important maintenance you do on your microscope is daily cleaning of the eyepieces, objectives, condenser and stage. Clean the lenses, oculars, and the glass surface of the condenser with lens paper only. Other materials, such as tissues or paper towels, are abrasive and will scratch the lenses. Commercially available lens cleaner or alcohol can be used to clean the glass surfaces of the microscope thoroughly. After cleaning the glass surface with a piece of lens paper saturated with either lens cleaner or alcohol, it is important to remove any residual cleaner with a clean, dry piece of lens paper. **Do not allow the lens cleaner to air dry on the glass surfaces.**
- Always focus the microscope using the low-power (4× or 10×) objective first; then turn to the high-power (40×) or oil-immersion (100×) objective.
- Do not use the coarse adjustment when the high-power or oil-immersion objective is in position.
- Before storing a microscope, always clean it thoroughly. Be sure to wipe all oil from the oil-immersion lens. The microscope should be stored with the low-power objective in position. It should also be covered to prevent dust from settling on the lenses.

CHAPTER 2 PRETEST ANSWERS

1. See Figure 2-2.

2. False. The microscope can compensate for differences in visual acuity. Therefore, it is best if eyeglasses are not worn when looking in the microscope.

3. False. The oil is placed on the top of the slide and provides a connection between the slide and the objective.

4. This is a true statement.

5. The correct answer is c. In a urine specimen cells are counted per high-power field.

CHAPTER 2 POSTTEST

1. Name the three objectives found on most clinical microscopes. Calculate the final magnification of each objective
   if the oculars provide 10× magnification.

2. Discuss how each of the above objectives would be used
   when looking at

   a. a slide of urine sediment.

   b. a Gram-stained smear.

3. Describe how the condenser and aperture diaphragm opening should be set when studying

   a. unstained wet-mount specimens.

   b. Gram-stained specimens.

4. Describe the functions of the following parts of the microscope:

   a. Condenser

   b. Oculars

   c. Mechanical stage

Question 5: Fill in the blank.

5. In microscopy, the ability to discern two points as distinct entities is called _____.

6. You are examining an unstained urine sediment. Regardless of the objective you are using, your field of focus is obscured by concentric gray rings that do not move when you move the slide. What is the most likely cause of this problem?

Question 7: Multiple choice. Select the one best answer.

7. Regarding the proper use and care of the microscope, which one of the following is the **least** accurate statement?

   a. A microscope should be stored with the low-power objective locked into position.

   b. In order to avoid scratching the lens surfaces, clean the lenses only with abrasive-free material, such as lens paper.

   c. To remove dirt or oil from the objectives, wipe the lens with lens paper that has been saturated with alcohol or lens cleaner and allow the alcohol or lens cleaner to evaporate off the lens.

   d. Always carry a microscope in an upright position by supporting the base of the microscope with one hand and holding the arm of the microscope with the other hand.

CHAPTER 2 POSTTEST ANSWERS

1. The three objectives found on most clinical microscopes are:
   a. Low-power or 10× objective, final magnification 10 times ocular (10) = 100×
   b. High-power or 40× objective, final magnification 40 times ocular (10) = 400×
   c. Oil-immersion or 100× objective, final magnification 100 times ocular (10) = 1000×.

2. a. A slide of urine sediment: The **low-power** objective is used to focus the microscope, to scan the slide to determine the overall quality of the specimen, and to quantitate the number of casts. The **high-power** objective is used to identify and quantitate cells, bacteria, fungus, and crystals in a urine sediment. The **oil-immersion** objective should not be used when looking at urine sediments or wet-mount specimens.
   b. A Gram-stained smear: The **low-power** objective is used to focus the microscope and to scan the slide to determine the overall quality of the specimen. The **high-power** objective is not used when looking at Gram stains. The **oil-immersion** objective is used to identify cells and bacteria in Gram-stained specimens.

3. a. Unstained wet-mount specimens: Condenser should be raised to a position just below the slide and the aperture diaphragm should be closed.
   b. Gram-stained specimens: Condenser should be raised to a position just below the slide. The aperture diaphragm should be opened.

4. a. The **condenser** focuses the light on the slide.
   b. The **oculars** are the eyepieces of the microscope. They also provide a fixed magnification, usually 10×.
   c. The **stage** is the surface on which the slide rests. A **mechanical** stage allows you to move the slide on the stage by turning knobs usually located on the right side of the microscope.

5. Resolution

6. The problem is most likely dirt (fingerprints) on the ocular lenses. To rectify the problem, clean the oculars with lens paper.

7. The correct answer is c. When using alcohol or lens cleaner to clean the glass surfaces of the microscope, you should remove the excess cleaner with a dry piece of lens paper. The cleaning solutions should not be allowed to dry on the lens surface.

SUGGESTED READINGS

Rubbi, C. P. (1994). *Light microscopy: Essential data.* New York: Wiley.
Smith, R. F. (1993). *Microscopy and photomicrography.* Boca Raton, FL: CRC Press.

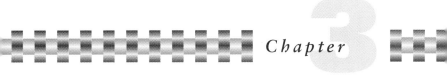

Urinalysis

The urinalysis is the most common laboratory test performed in a clinician's office. It is a relatively simple test to perform and can provide information about many different organ systems of the body (Table 3-1).

A urinalysis may be ordered as part of a routine physical examination, to monitor pregnant patients for toxemia and diabetes, to monitor patients with hypertension for renal disease, to manage diabetes, and to diagnose urinary tract infections.

OBJECTIVES

Upon completion of this chapter, the reader will be able to:

1. Describe the proper techniques for the collection of urine specimens for routine urinalysis and urine culture.
2. Describe the proper methods of handling urine specimens before analysis.
3. Perform a visual analysis of urine.
4. Perform a chemical analysis of urine.
5. Prepare urine sediment for microscopic analysis.
6. Examine urine sediment using a compound brightfield microscope.
7. Identify the following structures when viewed microscopically:
   - Epithelial cells
   - White blood cells
   - Red blood cells
   - Bacteria
   - Casts
   - Yeast

TABLE 3-1. Correlation of Urinalysis Results With Clinical Conditions

Clinical Condition	Dipstick Tests	Microscopic Findings
Carbohydrate metabolism	Glucose, ketone	
Kidney function	Protein, occult blood	Casts, RBCs, crystals
Liver function	Bilirubin, urobilonogen	Crystals
Urinary tract infection	Nitrite, blood, leukocyte esterase	WBCs, RBCs, bacteria, yeast, etc.
Acid-base balance	pH	
Dehydration/hydration	Specific gravity	

OBJECTIVES (Continued)

- Trichomonas
- Crystals

Please take the pretest. After completion of the pretest, read the material in the chapter.

CHAPTER 3 PRETEST

Questions 1–3: Multiple choice. Select the one best answer.

1. When microscopically examining a urine sediment, you should use the

   a. low-power objective.

   b. high-power objective.

   c. oil-immersion objective.

   d. a and b

   e. a and c

2. Terms commonly used to describe the visual appearance of a urine sample include all of the following **except:**

   a. Straw

   b. Milky

   c. Yellow

   d. Hazy

   e. Amber

3. Which of the following tests would **not** be performed as part of a routine urinalysis?

   a. Glucose

   b. Occult blood

   c. Microscopic examination for cells

   d. Determination of specific gravity

   e. Gram stain

Questions 4–6: Answer true or false.

4. For best results, urine specimens for routine analysis should be tested within 30 minutes of collection.

5. If bacteriologic culture is ordered, the urine specimen must be collected in a sterile container.

6. In the microscopic analysis, casts are counted per high-power field and appear as cylinders with dark, well-defined edges.

■ 7. Identify the cells in Figure 3–1 (400×).

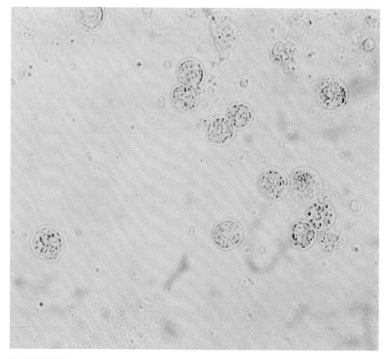

FIGURE 3-1
Pretest question #7 (400×).

■ *The pretest answers will appear throughout the text of the chapter and before the posttest.*

SPECIMEN COLLECTION

Specimen collection and handling are crucial components of any laboratory test. Stated another way, a laboratory test result is only as good as the specimen tested. This is especially true when testing urine specimens. An improperly collected or handled urine specimen can result in erroneous test results, leading to misdiagnosis and improper treatment.

Specimen Containers

Urine samples for routine urinalysis should be collected in clean disposable containers. Do not use homemade-type containers (eg, glass jars, pill bottles, etc.), because these containers may be contaminated with chemicals that will interfere with the urinalysis. For routine urinalysis, the container need not be sterile; if, however, bacteriologic culture is indicated or anticipated then the specimen must be collected in a sterile container.

▇ **Pretest question #5:** The following statement is true. If bacteriologic culture is ordered, the urine specimen must be collected in a sterile container.

Timing of Specimen Collection

The first-voided morning specimen is the most concentrated and, therefore, the preferred specimen for urinalysis. However, because it is often impractical to obtain the first morning specimen, randomly voided specimens are the most common specimens tested. The concentration of the urine (as measured by specific gravity) varies at different times of the day; therefore, when testing random specimens, the specific gravity should always be considered when interpreting results.

Methods of Collection

The preferred specimen for urinalysis is a clean-catch midstream (CCMS) urine specimen. Although not required for routine dipstick urinalysis, a CCMS specimen is required for urine culture and preferred for microscopic analysis. Therefore, to prevent having to request a second specimen for culture or microscopic exam, it is suggested that all urine testing be done on CCMS specimens. A properly collected CCMS urine specimen will contain fewer epithelial cells, mucous threads, and less genital contamination than non–clean-catch specimens.

COLLECTION OF CLEAN-CATCH MIDSTREAM URINE SPECIMENS

Patients should be given the appropriate collection materials and instructed on how to collect a proper CCMS urine specimen.
Collection materials:

1. Clean disposable specimen container (if urine culture is indicated, use a sterile container)
2. Two cleansing pads soaked with a mild antiseptic solution
3. One sterile dry pad or gauze.

Female Specimen Collection

1. Wash hands thoroughly.
2. Sit on the toilet and spread the labia with one hand. Use one of the cleansing pads provided (saturated with a mild antiseptic solution) to clean the urethral area by wiping the area in a front to back motion. Repeat this a second time using a clean pad. Wipe the area dry using sterile dry gauze.
3. With the labia still separated, release a small amount of urine into the toilet. The midstream portion of the urine is collected into the container provided. The final portion of the urine is voided into the toilet.

Male Specimen Collection

The procedure used for specimen collection in the male patient differs depending on the clinical situation.

If **cystitis** is suspected, a clean-catch, midstream specimen is collected.

1. Wash hands thoroughly.
2. Pull back the foreskin with one hand. Use one of the cleansing pads provided to clean the urethral opening. Repeat this a second time using a clean pad. Wipe the area dry using sterile dry gauze.
3. With the foreskin still retracted, release a small amount of urine into the toilet. The midstream portion of the urine is collected into the container provided. The final portion of the urine is voided into the toilet.

If **urethritis** is suspected, a voided specimen should be collected in the following manner:

1. Wash hands thoroughly.
2. Pull back the foreskin with one hand. Use one of the cleansing pads provided to clean the urethral opening. Repeat this a second time using a clean pad. Wipe the area dry using sterile dry gauze.
3. With the foreskin still retracted, collect the first 10 mL of urine in a container labeled as "first voided" or #1. This specimen is useful in the diagnosis of urethritis.

A midstream specimen is then collected in a second container labeled as "midstream" or #2. This specimen is useful in the diagnosis of cystitis.

If **prostatitis** is suspected, a third specimen should be collected in the following manner:

1. Wash hands thoroughly.
2. Pull back the foreskin with one hand. Use one of the cleansing pads provided to clean the urethral opening. Repeat this a second time using a clean pad. Wipe the area dry using sterile dry gauze.
3. With the foreskin still retracted, collect the first 10 mL of urine in a container labeled as "first voided" or #1. This specimen is useful in the diagnosis of urethritis. A midstream specimen is then collected in a second container labeled as "midstream" or #2. This specimen is useful in the diagnosis of cystitis. The patient is instructed not to empty the bladder completely.
4. While the patient continues to retract the foreskin, the clinician should massage the prostate with continuous strokes. If prostatic fluid is obtained, it should be collected in a sterile container for culture and Gram stain. This specimen should be labeled "expressed prostatic secretions" (EPS).
5. If fluid cannot be obtained, 10 mL of urine should be voided into a third sterile container (labeled "postmassage" or #3). This specimen represents approximately a 1:100 dilution of prostatic fluid and can be cultured, or centrifuged and stained to aid in the diagnosis of prostatitis.

OTHER METHODS OF COLLECTION

Catheterization.   This method carries the risk of introducing organisms into the bladder, which may, in turn, cause infection.

Suprapubic Aspiration.   This involves insertion of a needle directly into the bladder. This technique can be useful in obtaining specimens from infants.

Infant Bagged Specimen.   In order to obtain suitable specimens from infants and small children it is often necessary to use pediatric collection kits. These adhesive collection bags are attached to the genitalia. Care must be taken to remove the bag as soon as the sample is obtained. Also, specimens contaminated with fecal material should not be used for urinalysis.

One technique for obtaining pediatric specimens that is **not acceptable** for routine urinalysis is the practice of squeezing out diapers to obtain a specimen. These specimens contain abundant fibers and have essentially been filtered by the diaper material.

SPECIMEN HANDLING

Specimens should be examined within 30 minutes of collection. When specimens are left at room temperature, bacteria will multiply, utilizing any glucose present in the urine, which may alter the pH. Bilirubin and urobilinogen rapidly deteriorate, and casts and cellular elements decompose. If testing is to be delayed beyond 30 minutes, the best method for preserving the specimen is refrigeration at 5–8°C. Even with refrigeration, however, the specimen should be examined within 2 hours of collection. After refrigeration, the specimens should be allowed to return to room temperature before testing.

■ **Pretest question #4:** The following statement is true. For best results, urine specimens for routine analysis should be tested within 30 minutes of collection.

There are several commercially available urine preservatives that claim to preserve urine chemistries and cellular material.

Most of these products have some effect on one or more urine constituents. The package insert from these products will inform you of the results that may be affected by the preservative that is in use. If you use one of these products, be sure to be familiar with the recommendations from the manufacturer concerning how the product is to be used and if any of the results will be adversely affected by the preservative.

THE ROUTINE URINALYSIS

The routine urinalysis generally consists of three components:

1. Visual examination
2. Chemical examination using a reagent "dipstick"
3. Microscopic examination of urine sediment

■ **Pretest question #3:** The answer is e. The Gram stain is not part of a routine urinalysis.

Visual Examination

The physical characteristics of the urine specimen are color and turbidity.

COLOR

Terms commonly used to describe urine color include the following:

- Colorless (looks like water)
- Straw (pale yellow)
- Yellow
- Amber (reddish brown)
- Red
- Brown
- Green

Normal: Color varies with concentration, usually from straw to light amber.

TURBIDITY

Terms commonly used to describe urine turbidity include:

- Clear: No turbidity seen
- Hazy: Slight turbidity seen when the urine is held up to the light
- Cloudy: Obviously turbid, even before the urine is held up to the light
- Opaque: So turbid that print cannot be read through it

Normal: Clear

Pretest question #2: The answer is b. Milky is not a term that is used to describe the physical appearance of urine.

Chemical Examination

Chemical analysis of urine specimens is done using one of a number of commercially available "dipsticks." A dipstick is a narrow strip of plastic with small reagent pads attached to it. Each pad contains reagents for one chemical test. Up to 10 tests can be performed using one of the many strips that are commercially available. The tests on the strips include: bilirubin, blood, glucose, ketones, leukocyte esterase, nitrite, pH, protein, specific gravity, and urobilinogen.

Although relatively easy to use, one must remember that complex biochemical reactions are taking place on the reagent pads and, unless the strips are used properly, results cannot be relied upon. It is important to follow all manufacturer's directions when using the strips and to handle and store the strips properly.

There are several precautions that must be followed to ensure the accuracy of dipstick testing:

- Always perform dipstick testing on unspun urine that is at room temperature. If the specimen has been refrigerated, it should be allowed to return to room temperature before testing.
- Always read the reagent pads at the designated time after dipping the strip in the urine. These times are printed on the color charts and in the directions supplied with each bottle.

- Always keep the strips in the original container. Protect the strips from light, heat, and moisture. Store at room temperature away from any heat source.
- When removing strips, remove only the number you will need and quickly close the container, securing the cap tightly.
- The color of the reagent pads should be the same as the "negative" blocks on the color charts. Do not use the reagent pads if they are discolored.
- Do not use the strips after their expiration date. The expiration date is printed on the bottle.

It is beyond the scope of this book to discuss in detail the significance of the results of the various tests available on the dipsticks. The following section briefly discusses the 10 tests available on the dipsticks and the major clinical significance of those tests.

BILIRUBIN

The detection of increased amounts of bilirubin in the urine (**bilirubinuria**) is an early sign of liver disease or biliary obstruction. Normal: Negative

Bilirubinuria often occurs before any clinical signs of liver disease (jaundice, clinical illness) and therefore is an excellent diagnostic tool for liver disease.

Precaution: Bilirubin rapidly decomposes when exposed to heat or light, one important reason for rapid testing of fresh urine specimens.

BLOOD

Most dipstick tests for blood detect intact red blood cells (RBCs), free hemoglobin, and myoglobin. Normal: Negative

The presence of intact RBCs in the urine (**hematuria**) most likely indicates bleeding within the urinary tract. This may occur in a variety of renal disorders, urinary tract infections or tumors, trauma to the kidneys, viral infections, bleeding disorders, strenuous exercise, and menstrual contamination.

Free hemoglobin in the urine (**hemoglobinuria**) most often occurs as a result of lysis of RBCs within the urinary tract or after voiding. Lysis after voiding can occur in very dilute urine or very alkaline urine specimens.

True hemoglobinuria indicates intravascular hemolysis and occurs in such conditions as transfusion reactions, hemolytic anemias, severe burns, various poisonings and paroxysmal hemoglobinuria. If true hemoglobinuria is suspected, serum should be tested for hemoglobinemia. True hemoglobinuria should be suspected when the dipstick test for blood is positive, but the microscopic exam shows no RBCs or the degree of positive does not correlate with the number of RBCs present in the microscopic exam.

A positive dipstick test without the presence of RBCs in the microscopic exam may also indicate the presence of myoglobin in the urine (**myoglobinuria**). Myoglobinuria occurs in traumatic muscle injury.

GLUCOSE

Glucose is often present in the urine of individuals with diabetes mellitus. Normal: Negative

▓▓▓▓ Clinical Tip:

- Bacteria present in urine will metabolize glucose and can result in a falsely negative glucose result if the urine is allowed to stand at room temperature for longer than 30 minutes.

KETONES

Diabetes mellitus is the most important disorder in which ketones are found in the urine (**ketonuria**). If ketonuria occurs in an individual with diabetes, it is a sign that the disease is out of control and a change in insulin dosage or other changes in management are indicated. Ketonuria also occurs in conditions in which there is an inadequate dietary intake of carbohydrates. Examples include starvation, severe vomiting or diarrhea, fever, and certain gastrointestinal diseases. Normal: Negative

LEUKOCYTE ESTERASE

The leukocyte esterase test detects the presence of white blood cells (WBCs) in the urine sediment. The presence of a significant number of WBCs in the urine usually indicates a urinary tract infection. However, patients with genital tract infections (cervicitis, vaginitis, or urethritis) may also have WBCs in their urine. Normal: Negative

NITRITE

The nitrite test is an indirect indicator of bacteriuria (significant bacteria in the urine). Most of the organisms that cause urinary tract infections will reduce dietary nitrates to nitrites. The nitrites, if present, are detected by the dipstick.

▌▌▌ Clinical Tip

- Not all organisms that cause urinary tract infections will reduce nitrates (examples include Enterococcus and Staphylococcus) and therefore, false negative results can occur. Also, the urine must remain in the bladder for at least 4 hours for the bacteria to reduce the nitrates. This can be a problem because patients with urinary tract infections often experience the need to urinate frequently. Normal: Negative

pH

pH is a measure of the overall acid-base balance of the body and the kidneys' ability to regulate that balance. It is also important in the identification of crystals (see Fig. 3-22). Normal: 4.6–8.0

PROTEIN

Protein in the urine (**proteinuria**) is seen in a wide variety of disorders. Proteinuria is one of the most important indicators of renal dysfunction. It also occurs with high fevers, hypertension, toxemia in pregnancy, strenuous physical exercise, and emotional stress. Normal: Negative

SPECIFIC GRAVITY

The specific gravity is a measure of the amount of dissolved solutes in the urine; it therefore reflects the relative degree of concentration or dilution of the urine specimen. In the past, specific gravity was measured using a refractometer or urinometer. Today, a dipstick test for specific gravity is available and widely used. Normal: 1.003–1.030

Low specific gravity can be found in diabetes insipidus and various renal abnormalities. (Low specific gravity can be a normal finding in infants less than 3 months old.) High specific gravity can be found in hepatic disease, various renal abnormalities, and any condition that leads to dehydration (vomiting, diarrhea, fever, etc.).

The specific gravity is also important in the interpretation of other urine test results. For example, if a very dilute (low specific gravity) urine specimen contains 2–5 WBCs/HPF it may be clinically significant, whereas a similar finding in a more concentrated urine may be a normal finding.

UROBILINOGEN

Urinary urobilinogen is increased in hemolytic anemias, various liver diseases, malaria, and congestive heart failure.

Precaution: Urobilinogen rapidly decomposes when exposed to heat or light, which is one important reason for rapid testing of fresh urine specimens.

Normal: 0.2–1 mg/dL

Microscopic Examination

The microscopic exam is performed to detect elements or cells that do not give chemical reactions (eg, casts, epithelial cells, and crystals) and to confirm chemical test results— for example, seeing RBCs in a microscopic exam confirms a positive blood result. The microscopic and chemical results of a urinalysis should always be checked against each other and any discrepancies should be resolved before the results are reported. For example, a nitrite dipstick result of negative with a microscopic exam that shows many bacteria may indicate a urinary tract infection with an organism that does not reduce nitrates.

The microscopic examination should be done on the sediment from a centrifuged specimen. 10–15 mL of urine are placed in a centrifuge tube and spun at 2,500 RPMs for 5 minutes (See pp. 85–87 for instructions on how to use a centrifuge). After centrifugation, the supernatant is removed and a drop of the sediment is placed on a clean glass slide, coverslipped and viewed microscopically. More detailed instructions on preparation of the urine sediment and slides are in the section "Specimen Processing" (pp. 83–85).

There are stains available for urine sediments. The Sternheimer stain is very often used. There are advantages and disadvantages to the use of stains. Although they do make certain structures more visible and easier to identify, they also add to the cost of the procedure and may precipitate out, causing difficulty in reading the slide. Most practitioners prefer viewing unstained specimens; therefore, the examples shown here are of unstained specimens.

The reliability of the microscopic exam is dependent on the quality of the urine specimen and the ability of the person performing the examination. Regarding the quality of the specimen, urine should be examined as soon as possible after collection. The first morning specimen is preferred, as it is the most concentrated and usually acidic. However, random specimens are most commonly tested. When testing random specimens, keep in mind that those with low specific gravity or alkaline pH may lyse cells and casts.

Adequate training and experience are needed to become proficient at microscopy. This manual is merely an introduction to the many structures that may be present in a urine specimen. It is beyond the scope of this book to detail all the structures and cells that one might see in a urine sediment. The following pages will describe and illustrate the most common findings in urine sediments. Other than a good microscope, the most useful tool for performing microscopic urinalysis is a good urinary sediment atlas. It is very important to compare any unknown structures with pictures from an atlas for identification. The reference section of this book lists several excellent atlases that are currently available.

When viewing unstained urine sediments there are two important rules to follow.

1. The illumination of the microscope must be properly set. In order to achieve the appropriate contrast to see many of the

cells and structures, the aperture diaphragm must be closed when using the low-power (10×) objective. When magnification is increased to the high-power (40×) objective, the aperture diaphragm should be opened slightly until the optimal contrast is achieved.

2. Constantly turning the fine-focus adjustment knob on the microscope back and forth allows visualization of differences in density as well as different focal planes. Often, cells or structures will be in a slightly different focal plane. By using the fine-focus knob to change the focal plane, these cells or structures will come into focus.

▚▚▚ Clinical Tip

■ It is good practice to keep the fingers of your right hand on the stage travel-control knobs and the fingers of your left hand on the fine-focus adjustment knob. The slide is moved on the stage with your right hand and the fine-focus knob is turned back and forth with the left hand to better visualize the specimen.

COMMON MICROSCOPIC FINDINGS IN URINE SEDIMENT

EPITHELIAL CELLS: COUNTED PER HIGH-POWER FIELD (400X)

Squamous Epithelial Cells.   Large (30–50 μm), flat cells with a small central nucleus. They originate in the lower end of the urinary tract (distal third of the urethra) and, in females, the vagina. A large number of squamous epithelial cells in a urine sediment suggests contamination with urethral or vaginal secretions (Fig. 3-2).

Transitional Epithelial Cells.   Round or pear-shaped cell (20–30 μm) with a large central nucleus. They originate in the renal pelvis and upper 2/3 of the urethra. Normal in small numbers, but large numbers could be a sign of malignancy or recent instrumentation of the urinary tract (Fig. 3-3).

Renal Tubular Epithelial Cells.   Slightly smaller than transitional epithelial cells and may be cuboidal or columnar with a
(text continues on page 56)

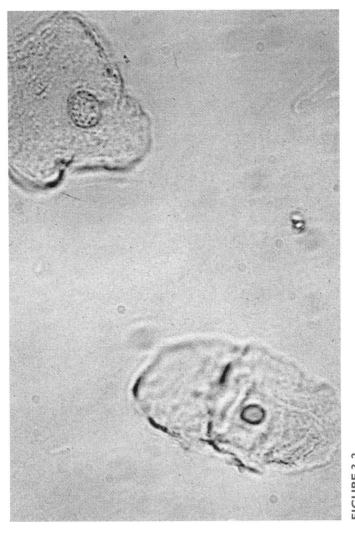

FIGURE 3-2
Squamous epithelial cell (400×).

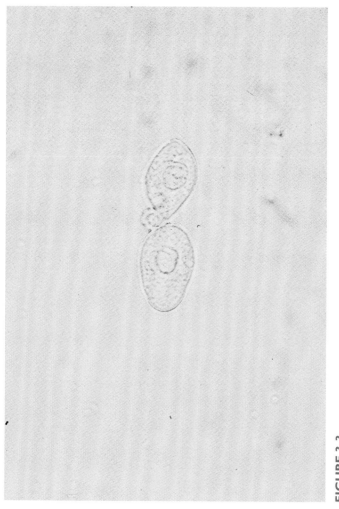

FIGURE 3-3
Transitional epithelial cell (500×).

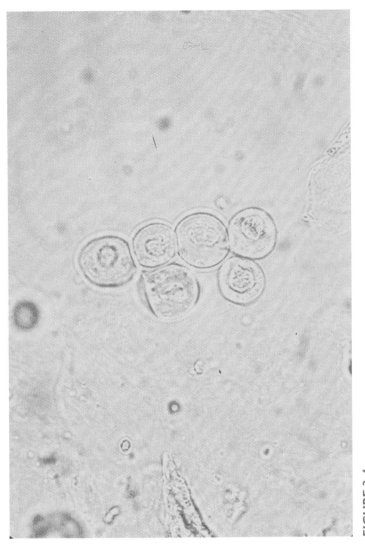

FIGURE 3-4
Renal tubular epithelial cell (500×).

large nucleus that may be slightly off center. It is often difficult to differentiate them from transitional cells. Small numbers may appear in normal urine. Increased numbers suggest tubular damage which may occur in patients on cancer chemotherapy, renal transplant patients, patients exposed to various toxins, or patients with various viral infections (Fig. 3-4).

BLOOD CELLS: COUNTED PER HIGH-POWER FIELD (400×)

Red Blood Cells (RBCs).   Normal: 0–3 per HPF.

In fresh urine, RBCs are pale, yellowish, smooth biconcave disks. They are 7–10 μm in size and do not have granules or a nucleus. They are very refractile and are thicker on the edges than in the center. When changing the focus, the red cells "pop out" at the viewer as black circles (Figs. 3-5 and 3-6).

In hypertonic urine, RBCs may shrink and develop a notched appearance, a process called crenation. Crenated RBCs may appear to have granules and thus be confused with WBCs. In Figure 3-6, note the RBCs that appear to have granules (arrows). These are spicules on the surface of crenated RBCs. In hypotonic urine, "ghost cells" cells may appear pale with little hemoglobin.

RBCs may be present in a variety of conditions. Hematuria is a common finding in urinary tract infections, renal disorders or tumors, trauma to the kidneys, viral infections, bleeding disorders, strenuous exercise, and menstrual contamination.

White Blood Cells (WBCs).   Normal: 3–5 per HPF.

The polymorphonuclear (poly, seg, PMN, neutrophil) cell is the most common WBC seen in the urine. It is 10–12 μm in size and has a multisegmented nucleus and granules present in the cytoplasm (Fig. 3-7; also see Fig. 3-5)

An increase in WBCs in the urine is called **pyuria**. The most common causes of pyuria in females is cystitis and vaginitis/cervicitis. In males, the most common causes of pyuria are urethritis and prostatitis. When interpreting the meaning of the presence of WBCs in a male urine specimen, it is important to know how the specimen was collected. This can help in determining whether the patient has cystitis, urethritis, or prostatitis (Table 3-2).

(text continues on page 60)

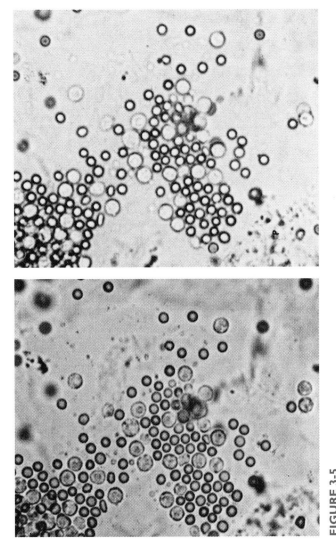

FIGURE 3-5
Red and white blood cells (400×). Note that a slight change of focus causes the red cells to appear as black circles.

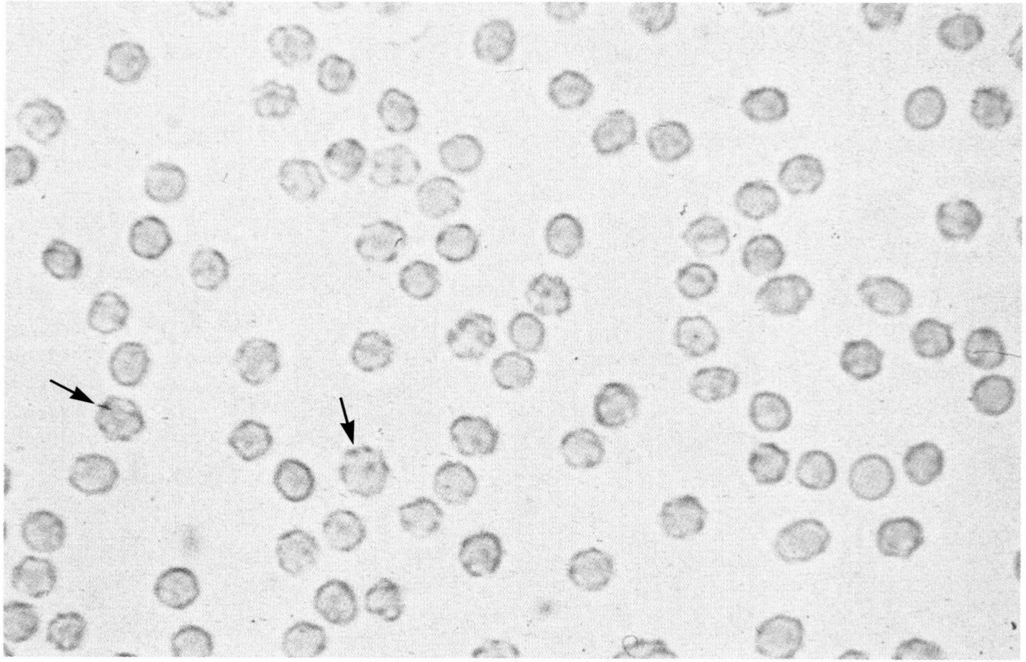

FIGURE 3-6
Red blood cells. Arrows indicate crenated cells (400×).

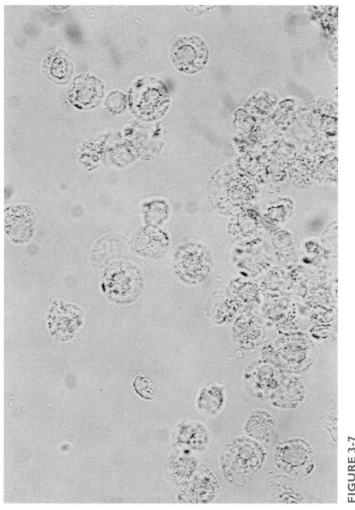

FIGURE 3-7
White blood cells (800X). *Note:* These cells have been enlarged to show detail.

TABLE 3-2. Relative Numbers of White Blood Cells in Specimen

	Specimen #1: First Voided	Specimen #2: Midstream	Specimen #3: Post–prostatic massage
Cystitis	+	+	+
Urethritis	+ +	±	±
Prostatitis	+	+	+ +

CASTS: COUNTED PER LOW-POWER FIELD (100×)

Casts are cylindrically shaped elements that are formed in the tubular portion of the kidneys and excreted in the urine. They are composed of a protein matrix that may or may not contain cells or other elements. Because the protein matrix has a very low refractive index, it is very hard to see in an unstained specimen. (The aperture diaphragm must be closed in order to obtain the contrast necessary to see casts.) Casts have parallel sides and rounded or blunted ends. Casts vary in length and width and **do not have dark edges.** Any structure that has dark, thick edges is most likely a fiber of some sort and not a cast.

Casts are categorized according to their content and morphologic characteristics and are reported as the type and the number per low-power (100×) field.

■ **Pretest question #6:** The following statement is false. In the microscopic analysis of urine, casts are counted per high-power field and appear as cylinders with dark, well-defined edges.

Hyaline Casts. Hyaline casts are composed of the protein matrix without any inclusions. They are colorless, homogenous, and transparent. This makes them very difficult to see and illustrates the importance of having the condenser and aperture diaphragm set correctly (Fig 3-8 A and B).

Hyaline casts are found in even the mildest forms of renal disease and are not associated with any one disease. A few hyaline casts may be found in normal urine and increased numbers may be seen following strenuous physical exercise (may be increased for 24 hours).

Granular Casts. Granular casts may be the result of the degeneration of cellular casts, or they may represent the aggregation of serum proteins within the protein matrix. Whatever the origin, the surface of these casts look like fine or coarse sandpaper. They are much easier to see than hyaline casts because of the granules within the protein matrix. Granular casts are divided into fine and coarse granular casts on the basis of the size of the granules within the cast (Fig. 3-9).

Granular casts are seen in many renal diseases and usually indicate significant renal disease. However, small numbers may be seen following strenuous physical exercise.

Broad Waxy Casts. Highly refractive broad, short casts with blunt or broken ends. They often have cracked or serrated edges. Waxy casts are found in chronic renal failure (Fig. 3-10).

Red Blood Cell Casts. Casts in which RBCs are caught in the protein matrix. Distinct RBCs must be seen within the cast in order to identify it as an RBC cast. RBC casts are always clinically significant. They are generally diagnostic of glomerular disease, but, in rare instances, may be found in other conditions (Fig. 3-11).

White Blood Cell Casts. Casts in which WBCs are caught in the protein matrix. WBCs (mostly polymorphonuclear cells) must be seen within the cast in order to identify it as an WBC cast. WBC casts are seen in many renal disorders and are always clinically significant (Fig. 3-12 A and B).

Epithelial Cell Casts. Casts in which renal tubular epithelial cells are present in the protein matrix. Epithelial cell casts are seen in diseases that destroy the tubular epithelium, such as certain viral infections, and exposure to toxins (mercury, chemotherapeutic agents, salicylates [Fig. 3-13]).

Miscellaneous Casts. Other materials that may be trapped in the protein matrix of a cast include the following:

- Fat droplets—fatty cast
- Bile pigments—bile cast
- Hemoglobin pigments—hemoglobin cast
- Bacteria—bacterial cast

Figures of these casts and their clinical significance can be found in the suggested references or atlases.

(text continues on page 67)

FIGURE 3-8
(A) Hyaline casts (200×).

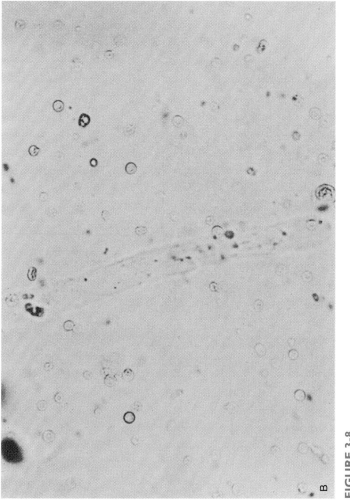

FIGURE 3-8
(**B**) Hyaline cast and red blood cell (400×).

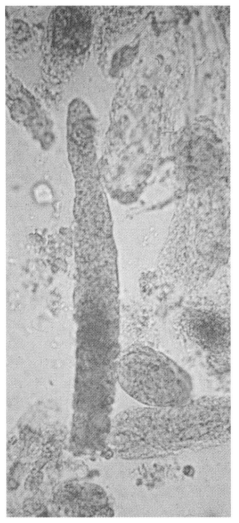

FIGURE 3-9
Granular casts (400×).

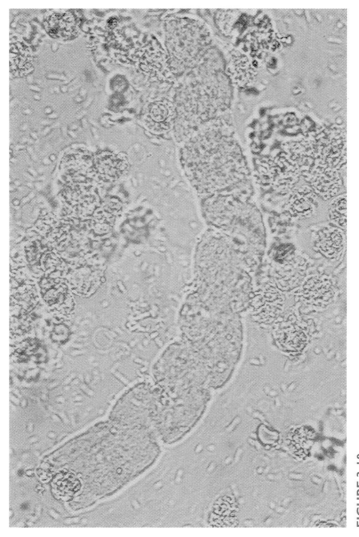

FIGURE 3-10
Broad waxy cast (500×).

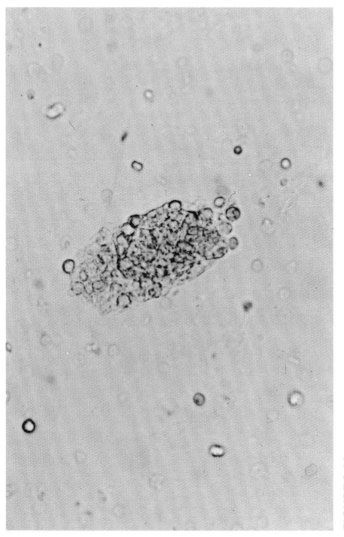

FIGURE 3-11
Red blood cell cast (400×).

MISCELLANEOUS STRUCTURES

Fibers. As mentioned earlier, casts have very fine edges. Structures resembling casts in size and shape that have dark edges are most likely fibers. Fibers also tend to be flat, whereas casts are cylindrical. Fibers may come from a variety of sources including clothing, diapers, toilet paper, or lint (Fig. 3-14).

Starch Granules. Starch granules are frequently found in the urine. The most common type seen in urine is cornstarch because many brands of powder contain cornstarch. Also, if powdered gloves are used, the slide or urine specimen may be accidentally contaminated with powder from the gloves. Starch granules are hexagonal in shape and have irregular indentations in the center (Fig. 3-15).

Bacteria. The shape and characteristics of individual organisms are best determined by doing a Gram stain (see Chapter 5). You can, however, using the 40X objective, see bacteria in a urine sediment as small, translucent organisms that may be round (cocci) or rod-shaped (rods). They may or may not be motile (Fig. 3-16).

If a properly collected, fresh urine specimen contains large numbers of bacteria (**bacteriuria**) and increased numbers of white blood cells, it is usually indicative of a urinary tract infection. On the other hand, if large numbers of bacteria are seen without white blood cells, the specimen may have been improperly collected or allowed to sit at room temperature too long.

Yeast. Yeast cells are smooth, oval cells with refractile walls. They may be approximately the same size and shape as red blood cells and therefore must be differentiated from them. Yeasts reproduce by a process called budding. A small daughter cell develops and eventually breaks off the mother cell. If a spherical or oval cell shows budding, then it is a yeast cell and not a red blood cell (Fig. 3-17).

Candida albicans is the most common yeast found in the urine. Yeast may cause urinary tract infections, especially in diabetic patients. Small numbers of yeast may also be present as a result of skin or vaginal contamination of the urine.

Trichomonas Vaginalis. *Trichomonas vaginalis* are spherical or pear-shaped parasites that are slightly larger than a white blood cell (15–20 μm). The characteristic most needed for the identifica-
(text continues on page 75)

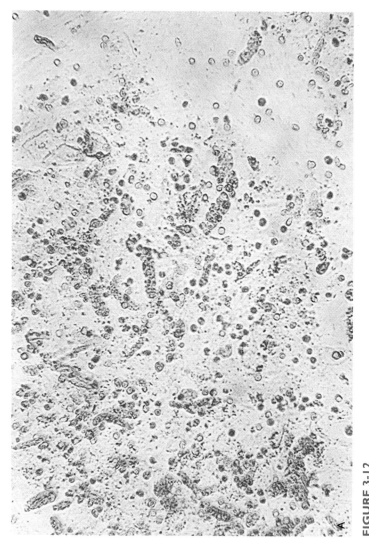

FIGURE 3-12
(A) Many white blood cells and white blood cell casts (200×).

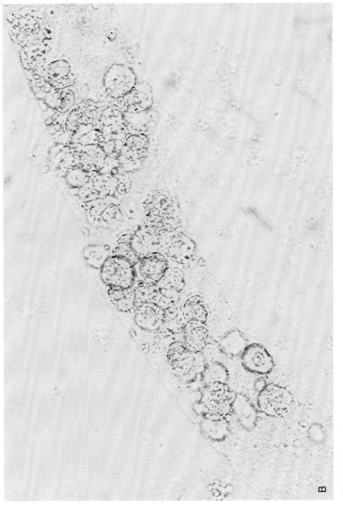

FIGURE 3-12
(B) White blood cell cast (500×).

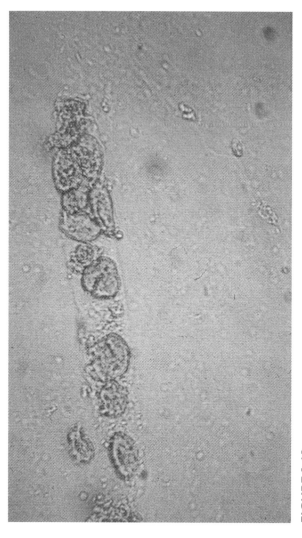

FIGURE 3-13
Epithelial cell cast (400×).

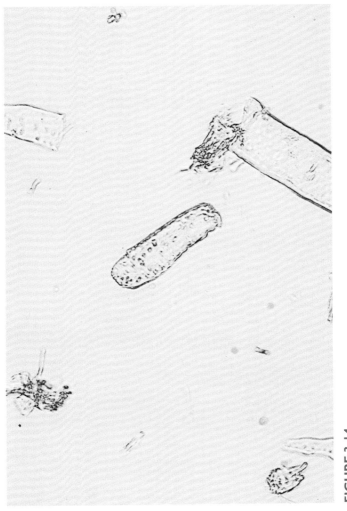

FIGURE 3-14
Fibers (400×); note dark edges.

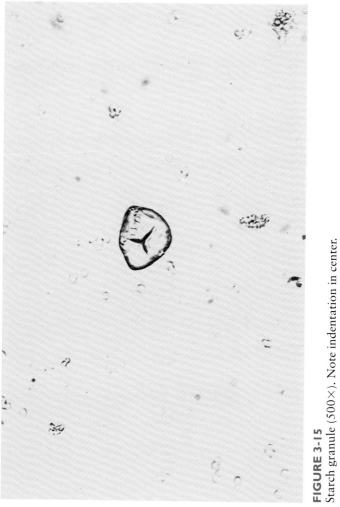

FIGURE 3-15
Starch granule (500×). Note indentation in center.

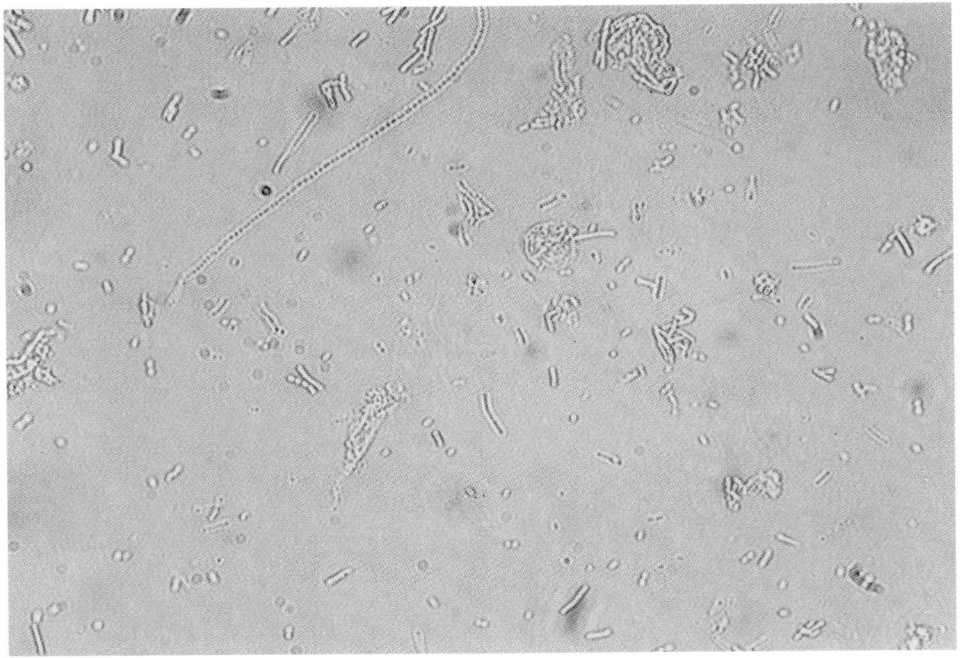

FIGURE 3-16
Bacteria (500×).

FIGURE 3-17
Budding yeast (400×).

tion of *T. vaginalis* is motility. Nonmotile organisms can easily be confused with WBCs or transitional epithelial cells. Therefore it is crucial that the characteristic motility of these organisms be seen in order to confirm their identification (Fig. 3-18).

Spermatozoa.   Sperm may be found in the urine of both sexes. Sperm have small oval bodies and long, thin tails (Fig. 3-19).

Mucus Threads.   Mucus is a normal finding in urine specimens, but increased amounts may indicate inflammation of the urinary tract. Mucus threads appear as ribbonlike structures that may be confused with hyaline casts. Mucus threads have approximately the same density as hyaline casts, but mucus threads generally do not have the parallel sides or cylindrical shape of hyaline casts. Also, unlike hyaline casts, they have pointed or frayed edges (Fig. 3-20).

Oil Droplets.   Oil droplets are a common contaminate of urine specimens. They are spherical and can vary greatly in size (Fig. 3-21).

CRYSTALS

Crystals are not usually found in freshly voided urine but appear after the urine stands for awhile. Many of the crystals found in the urine have little clinical significance except in cases of metabolic disorders, calculus formation, and the regulation of medication.

Crystal formation tends to be pH dependent. In order to identify a crystal present in a urine sample, it is important to know the pH of the urine.

Figure 3-22 is a guide to the identification of crystals. It is not complete nor meant to be a reference. It is merely an introduction to the most commonly seen crystals or crystals with particular clinical significance. It is highly recommended that a urinary sediment atlas be purchased and used for the identification of any unusual crystals found in a specimen.

Crystals in Acid Urine

Uric acid: Polymorphic in size and shape: diamond, rhombic prism and rosette. Usually stained with urinary pigments and, therefore, yellow or red-brown in color. Considered pathologic only when they appear in freshly voided specimens. Pathology in-

(text continues on page 82)

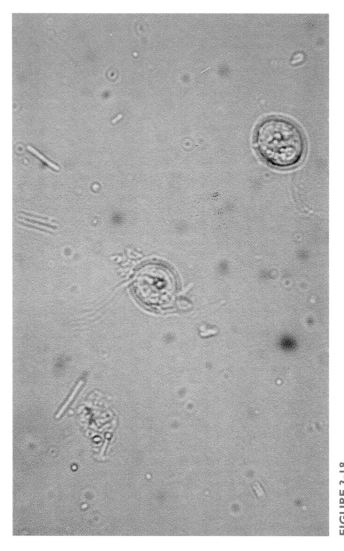

FIGURE 3-18
Trichomonas (1000×). *Note:* Organism is enlarged.

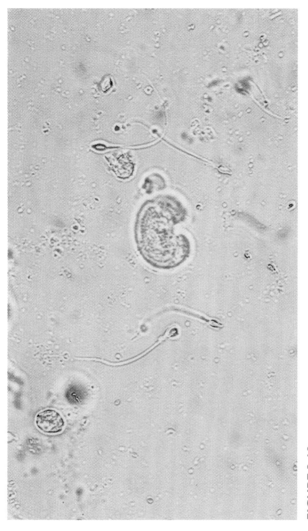

FIGURE 3-19
Sperm (500×).

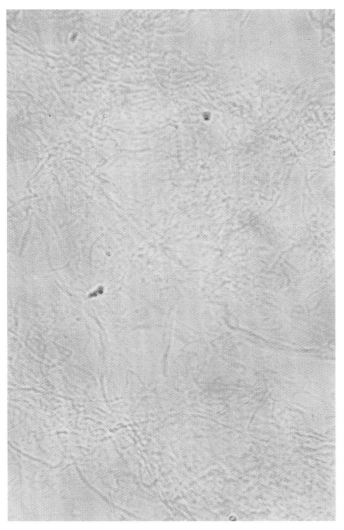

FIGURE 3-20
Mucus threads (100×).

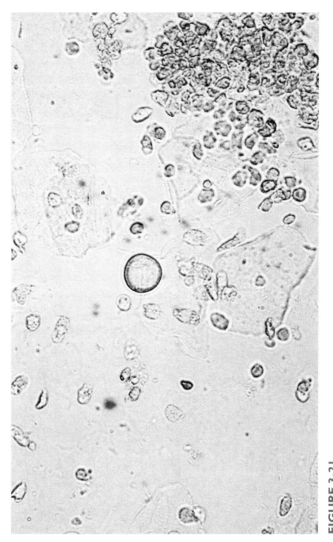

FIGURE 3-21
Oil droplet, white blood cells, and squamous epithelial cells (400×).

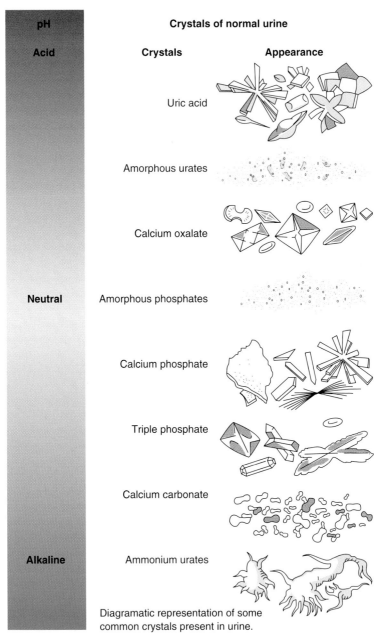

pH

Acid

Neutral

Alkaline

Crystals of normal urine

Crystals   **Appearance**

Uric acid

Amorphous urates

Calcium oxalate

Amorphous phosphates

Calcium phosphate

Triple phosphate

Calcium carbonate

Ammonium urates

Diagramatic representation of some
common crystals present in urine.

FIGURE 3-22
Crystals that may be found in urine sediment. Reprinted with permission
from M.H. Haber. (1991) *A primer of microscopic urinalysis* (2nd ed.).
Garden Grove, CA: Hycor Biomedical Inc.

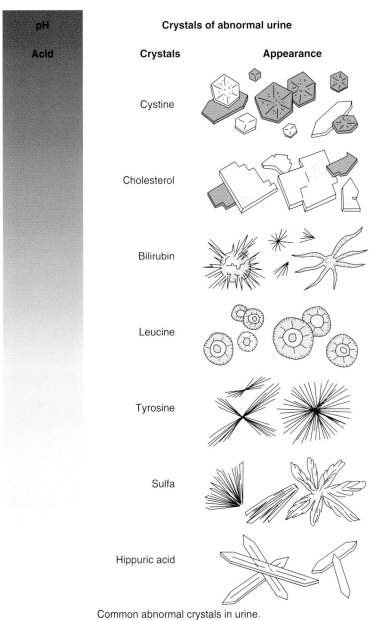

pH	Crystals of abnormal urine	
Acid	Crystals	Appearance
	Cystine	
	Cholesterol	
	Bilirubin	
	Leucine	
	Tyrosine	
	Sulfa	
	Hippuric acid	

Common abnormal crystals in urine.

FIGURE 3-22

cludes gout, acute febrile conditions, and certain chronic renal diseases. Presence of these crystals is of no significance in specimens that have cooled.

Amorphous urates: Salts of uric acid. Precipitates in urine specimens that have been refrigerated or cooled. Pink, tan, or yellowish red. Cleared by suspending sediment in warm saline and recentrifuging.

Calcium oxalate: Colorless octahedral or "envelope" shaped crystals. Present after ingestion of oxalate-rich foods (tomatoes, asparagus, spinach, garlic). Large amount may indicate oxalate calculi. Also found in diabetes mellitus, liver disease, and large doses of vitamin C.

Hippuric acid: Yellow-brown or colorless elongated prisms, no significance.

Cystine: Colorless, refractile, hexagonal plates. Found in patients with disorder of amino acid metabolism.

Leucine: Oily, highly refractile yellow or brown spheroids with radial concentric striations. Found in patients with maple syrup urine disease or serious liver disease (terminal cirrhosis and viral hepatitis). Often found together with tyrosine crystals.

Tyrosine: Fine, highly refractile needles occurring in sheaves or clusters. Found in patients with disorder of amino acid metabolism.

Cholesterol: Large, flat, transparent plates with notched corners. Indicates excessive tissue breakdown; can be seen in various renal diseases.

Sulfa: Highly refractile needles or sheaves; may be fan shaped, colorless to yellowish brown. Rarely found. May be seen in the urine of patients taking certain sulfa drugs.

Crystals in Alkaline Urine

Triple phosphate: Colorless prisms with 3–6 sides, frequently having oblique ends or "coffin lids." Usually no significance.

Amorphous phosphates: Fine, white granular crystals. They may obscure other elements in the urine sediment. Amorphous phosphates are soluble in dilute acetic acid and may be cleared by adding a drop of acetic acid to the urine sediment. No clinical significance.

Calcium carbonate: Small, colorless, "dumbbell" shaped granules. No clinical significance.

Calcium phosphate: Colorless crystals appearing as granules, rosettes, or large, flat irregularly shaped crystals. Usually no significance.

Ammonium biurates: Yellow-brown irregular crystals with radiating spicules, "thorn apples." No clinical significance.

SPECIMEN PROCESSING

This section describes the procedure for doing a complete urinalysis. To date, there has not been standardization of the urinalysis test procedure. Different laboratories may have procedures that vary slightly from the one described below. When performing any laboratory test, it is important to have a written procedure and to follow that procedure each time a test is done. For example, a laboratory may centrifuge 15 mL of urine at 2,000 RPM. This is an acceptable procedure as long as all urine specimens in that laboratory are tested using those same parameters.

1. After collection, mix the urine sample and decant approximately 12 mL of urine into a centrifuge tube. Note: If the urine has been refrigerated, it must be warmed to room temperature before testing.
2. Examine the urine for color and turbidity. Record the results.
3. Remove one urine dipstick from the bottle (immediately replace bottle cap) and dip it into the centrifuge tube, being sure that all the reagent pads are covered with urine. Note the exact time.
4. Immediately remove the dipstick from the urine. Remove excess urine by running the edge of the dipstick along the opening of the tube.
5. Hold the dipstick horizontally alongside the color chart on the dipstick bottle and carefully match the colors at the appropriate times.
6. Record the dipstick test results.
7. Place the specimen tube in the centrifuge. **Be sure centrifuge is balanced before spinning your urine specimen.**

Centrifuge for 5 minutes at 2,500 rpm. (See pp. 85–87 for instructions on how to use a centrifuge).

8. After the centrifuge has come to a **complete stop**, remove the specimen tube.

9. Decant the centrifuged urine tube by *quickly* inverting the tube over the sink. Turn the centrifuge tube over completely and let all the urine decant out of the tube.

10. After all the urine has decanted out of the centrifuge tube, turn the tube right side up and allow the urine that has clung to the sides of the tube to flow down to the bottom of the centrifuge tube. About 0.5 mL of urine will remain in the tube along with any sediment.

11. Mix the sediment by holding the top of the tube with the thumb and index finger and tapping the bottom of the tube with the index finger of the opposite hand.

12. Using a plastic pipette place 1 drop of the well-mixed sediment on a clean microscope slide.

13. Carefully place a coverslip over the drop. To avoid getting air bubbles, hold the coverslip with your thumb and forefinger perpendicular to the drop of sediment. Release the coverslip so that it falls directly on the drop of sediment. The presence of a few air bubbles, however, is not a disaster; just avoid looking at those areas when viewing the slide. Many air bubbles will cause the specimen to dry out too rapidly. When the coverslip is placed on the drop of urine, the liquid should fill the area under the coverslip. However, the urine should not overflow to the area of the slide outside the coverslip. Slide preparations with too little liquid will dry out too rapidly and slide preparations with too much liquid may be too thick to view adequately or may contaminate the microscope objective.

14. Raise the condenser to just below the slide and close the aperture diaphragm on the microscope. Place the slide on the microscope stage and focus using the low-power (10X) objective.

15. Move the stage until the edge of the coverslip is in view. Examine the area around the four sides of the coverslip. Remember to move the fine-adjustment knob back and forth constantly. Look carefully for casts, which are frequently found along the edges of the coverslip. If casts are seen, report the number per low-power field (LPF). To identify the type of cast, switch to the high-power (40×) objective.

16. Scan the rest of the coverslipped area under low power to get a general impression of the specimen.
17. Switch to the high-power objective. The light may need to be increased by opening the aperture diaphragm slightly. Examine 5–10 fields. Count the number of cells you see in each field. RBCs, WBCs, and epithelial cells are enumerated per high-power field. Example: 5–10 WBCs per HPF. TNTC = too numerous to count.

Use 1+ to 4+ for bacteria, mucus, yeast, sperm, amorphous material, and crystals.

1+ occasional
2+ noted in every field
3+ moderate to large amount in every field
4+ full or obscured field

■ **Pretest question #1:** The answer is d. Both the low-power and high-power objectives are used to microscopically examine urine sediment.

HOW TO USE A CENTRIFUGE

A centrifuge is an instrument that separates different elements within a sample on the basis of differences in the densities of those elements. There are many different kinds of centrifuges, from the very simple to the very complex. The manufacturer of the centrifuge must provide detailed instructions on the use and maintenance of each type of centrifuge, and these instructions should be followed to ensure accurate test results and safety in the laboratory. In general, the following applies to the use of all centrifuges.

1. The centrifuge should be placed on a level, stable surface. It should not be placed close to microscopes or other sensitive instruments, because the vibrations from the centrifuge may interfere with other equipment.
2. It is essential that the centrifuge be balanced. This means that the two tubes that are directly across from each other must have approximately the same weight. For example, in Figure 3-23, the centrifuge tube that is put into holder #1 in the centrifuge must weigh the same as the tube in holder #4.

It is not necessary to weigh the tubes when centrifuging urine specimens. If the tubes are the same size, from the same manufacturer, and contain the same amount of fluid, then their weights are close enough for these relatively slow centrifuges. In other words, if centrifuge tube #1 contains 12 mL of urine, then centrifuge tube #4 must contain 12 mL of urine. If tube #2 contains 10 mL of urine, then tube #5 must contain 10 mL of urine, and so on (see Fig. 3-23).

3. If an odd number of specimens is being spun, the centrifuge can be balanced by using a tube containing a volume of water equal to the specimen tube opposite.

4. If the centrifuge is not balanced properly, it will make loud noises and bounce on the counter surface. Should this happen, immediately turn off the centrifuge.

5. Centrifuge tubes should have tops, and specimens should be spun with the tops in place. This prevents the creation of potentially infectious aerosols.

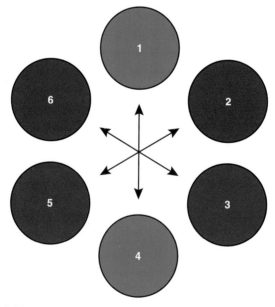

FIGURE 3-23
Balancing a centrifuge.

6. Do not open the lid of the centrifuge until it has come to a full and complete stop. Never try to slow down the centrifuge with your finger, a pencil, or any other item.
7. Be sure to keep the centrifuge clean. The inside of the centrifuge should be cleaned daily with a disinfectant. Also, be sure to disinfect the centrifuge adequately if a spill occurs.

QUALITY CONTROL

CLIA '88 regulations set specific quality-control parameters for laboratory testing. The quality-control requirements are dependent on the complexity category of the test procedure.

Urine Dipstick Analysis (Waived Test)

The quality-control requirements for waived tests are to follow the manufacturer's instructions for performing the test and quality-control measures.

Urine dipsticks should be tested with known positive and negative controls, which are available from different manufacturers. It is essential to do control testing when a new bottle of dipsticks is first opened. Additionally, how often to run the controls must be established by each laboratory. Daily control testing is preferred; however, if stored properly, urine dipsticks are very stable and weekly control testing may be adequate.

Microscopic Analysis (Moderate Complexity Test—Subcategory PPM)

Laboratories performing PPM tests must adhere to the quality-control standards of laboratories performing moderate complexity tests. These standards are published in the CLIA '88 regulations, subpart K. An important component of the quality-control requirements is that there must be a written procedure manual and "written quality control procedures for monitoring and evaluating the quality of the analytical testing process of each method to assure the accuracy and reliability of patient test results and reports" (Federal Register, 1992, p. 7163).

Because the microscopic examination of urine is a subjective, semiquantitative analysis, it is difficult to control adequately with objective, quantitative control reagents. Perhaps the most important measure to ensure accuracy of test results is proper training of all personnel performing a microscopic urinalysis. Also, reference materials and atlases should be readily available for comparison of any unknown structures that may be encountered when doing a microscopic exam of urine. The reference section of this chapter has several recommended urine sediment atlases that are currently available.

CHAPTER 3 PRETEST ANSWERS

1. The answer is d. Both the low-power and high-power objectives are used to examine a urine specimen microscopically.

2. The answer is b. Milky is not a term that is used to describe the physical appearance of a urine specimen.

3. The answer is e. A Gram stain is not part of a routine urinalysis.

4. True

5. True

6. False. Casts are counted per low-power field and do not have dark edges.

7. The cells are white blood cells. See Figure 3-7.

CHAPTER 3 POSTTEST

1. Name the three components of a routine urinalysis.

2. What is the preferred method for preserving a urine specimen if analysis must be delayed?

Questions 3–5: Multiple choice. Select the one best answer.

3. Regarding dipstick testing of urine, which one of the following statements is **least** accurate?

   a. Dipstick testing of urine should be done before the specimen is centrifuged for microscopic analysis.

   b. Dipsticks can be inactivated by heat, light, and moisture. Therefore, it is important to replace the cap on the bottle quickly and always store the dipsticks in the original bottle.

   c. Reading of the dipstick results can be done any time after the designated time on the reagent bottle, but never before the stated time. This is because, after the designated time, the reaction is stable and will not change over time.

   d. A positive and negative control specimen should be run every time a new bottle of dipsticks is opened.

4. Regarding the microscopic analysis of urine, which one of the following statements is **least** accurate?

   a. Microscopic analysis is done on the sediment from centrifuged urine specimens.

   b. Red blood cells and white blood cells are counted using the high-power objective, whereas casts are counted using the low-power objective.

   c. Casts are structures composed of a protein matrix that are often found around the edges of the coverslip.

   d. To identify bacteria adequately in a urine sediment, the oil-immersion objective should be used.

5. Regarding the collection of urine specimens, which one of the following statements is **least** accurate?

   a. Because the first morning specimen is more concentrated than a random specimen, it is preferred for doing a routine urinalysis.

   b. Specimens that may require bacteriologic culture should be collected by the clean-catch midstream method into a sterile container.

   c. To obtain a specimen from an infant for routine urinalysis carefully observe the infant; immediately after the infant voids into his/her diaper remove the diaper and wring it out into a urine specimen container.

   d. Catheterization should be used only when necessary because inserting the catheter can lead to seeding the bladder with bacteria which can result in a urinary tract infection.

Questions 6–7: *Fill in the blank.*

6. Figure 3-24 represents several microscopic fields of a urine specimen. The urinary element present in abnormal numbers can be classified as _____.

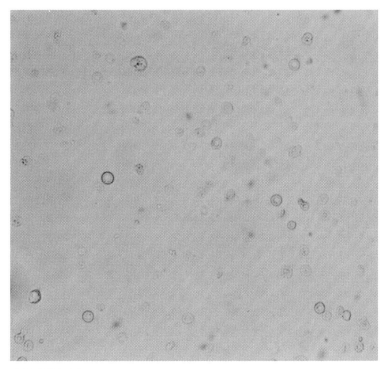

FIGURE 3-24
Posttest question #6 (400×).

7. The structure in Figure 3-25 is most likely
   _____.

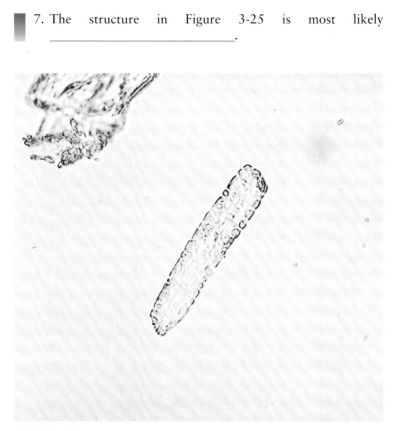

FIGURE 3-25
Posttest question #7 (400×).

CHAPTER 3 POSTTEST ANSWERS

1. Macroscopic examination, chemical examination, and microscopic examination

2. Refrigeration at 4°C

3. The least accurate statement is c. Reading of the dipsticks must be done precisely at the stated time. Reactions are not reliable after the stated time.

4. The least accurate statement is d. Bacteria can be seen with the 40X objective. The oil objective should not be used when looking at urine sediment.

5. The least accurate statement is c. This is an unacceptable method for obtaining a urine specimen from an infant. Special pediatric collection bags are available and should be used for pediatric urine collection.

6. Red blood cells

7. Fiber

REFERENCES

Clinical Laboratory Improvement Amendments of 1988, final rule. 42 CFR Part 405, et al. *Federal Register*, (Feb. 28 1992). 7,002–7,186.
Haber, M. H. (1991). *A primer of microscopic urinalysis* (2nd ed.). Garden Grove, CA: Hycor Biomedical Inc.

SUGGESTED READINGS AND URINARY ATLASES

Free, H. M. (ed.) (1996). *Modern urine chemistry*. Tarrytown, NY: Bayer Corporation, Diagnostics Division.
Graff, L. (1983). *A handbook of routine urinalysis*. Philadelphia: J. B. Lippincott.
Haber, M. H. (1991). *Urinary sediment: A textbook atlas*. Chicago: American Society of Clinical Pathologists.
Ringsrud, K. M., & Linné, J. J. (1995). *Urinalysis and body fluids: A colortext and atlas*. St. Louis: Mosby.

Diagnosis of Vaginitis/Vaginosis

Vaginitis is an inflammation of the vaginal mucosa and can present with a variety of symptoms, including vaginal discharge, malodor, irritation, burning or itching, dysuria, and dyspareunia. Two organisms that frequently cause vaginitis are *Candida albicans* and *Trichomonas vaginalis*. These organisms cause an inflammatory response; as a consequence, an increased number of white blood cells (polymorphonuclear cells) can be found in vaginal secretions.

Similar symptoms may be seen in the condition vaginosis. In this condition, however, there is no inflammatory response and, thus, white blood cells are not a prominent finding. The two most common types of vaginosis are bacterial vaginosis and cytolytic vaginosis.

Effective treatment of vaginitis/vaginosis depends upon an accurate identification of the cause of the symptoms. In deciding how to treat a patient with vaginitis/vaginosis, practitioners have relied on history, physical examination, vaginal pH, and microscopic examinations of vaginal secretions. The microscopic examinations include a saline wet mount and potassium hydroxide (KOH) preparation.

It is important to remember that patients complaining of vaginal discharge or symptoms of vaginitis/vaginosis may have cervicitis. Therefore, patients should also be evaluated for cervicitis. Chapter 6 discusses methods for obtaining endocervical specimens for laboratory analysis.

OBJECTIVES

Upon completion of this chapter, the reader will be able to:

1. Describe the proper technique for the collection and handling of vaginal secretions.
2. Determine the pH of vaginal secretions.
3. Perform a saline wet-mount analysis on vaginal secretions.
4. Perform a KOH analysis on vaginal secretions.
5. Recognize the following when viewed microscopically:
   - Epithelial cells
   - "Clue" cells
   - White blood cells
   - Red blood cells
   - Bacteria, including lactobacilli
   - Yeast
   - Trichomonas
6. Correlate laboratory and clinical findings to diagnose the causes of vaginitis/vaginosis.

Please take the pretest. After completing the pretest, read the material in the chapter.

CHAPTER 4 PRETEST

Questions 1–3: Multiple choice: Select the one best answer.

1. The "whiff" test is used in the diagnosis of:

   a. Candidiasis

   b. Bacterial vaginosis

   c. Trichomoniasis

   d. Gonorrhea

   e. Cervicitis

2. The KOH preparation of a vaginal discharge is used to identify:

   a. Fungal elements

   b. Trichomonads

   c. Bacteria

   d. "Clue cells"

   e. White blood cells

3. When analyzing a wet mount of a vaginal discharge, all the following cells or organisms may be observed **except:**

   a. *Candida albicans*

   b. *Neisseria gonorrhoeae*

   c. *Trichomonas vaginalis*

   d. "Clue cells"

   e. White blood cells

Questions 4–6: *Answer true or false.*

4. It is best to examine a vaginal wet-mount specimen soon after collection. However, if a delay is anticipated, refrigerate the specimen to maintain cellular integrity.

5. The saline wet mount is examined using both the low-power and high-power objectives.

6. Multiple infections are not uncommon. Therefore be sure to examine the wet-mount specimen fully even if one cause for the vaginitis is quickly ascertained.

The pretest answers will appear throughout the text of the chapter and before the posttest.

SALINE WET-MOUNT PREPARATION

The saline wet-mount preparation is a direct, rapid test for the identification of cells and microorganisms most commonly associated with vaginitis. With this test, one can detect the presence of bacteria and identify cells (WBCs, RBCs, epithelial, and clue cells), yeast and pseudohyphae, and motile *Trichomonas*.

Specimen Collection and Slide Preparation

Some clinicians prepare the saline wet mount and KOH mount by placing the specimen directly onto a slide at the time of the vaginal examination. This method is not recommended, because the slide often dries out before the clinician has a chance to examine it. A more appropriate method of specimen collection and processing is described below.

1. Place 1 mL of normal saline into a test tube. Label the test tube with the patient's name.
2. Insert vaginal speculum that has been moistened with warm **water** into the patient's vagina. Any lubricant other than water may interfere with slide analysis.
3. Expose the cervix and vaginal mucosa with the speculum and note the appearance of the mucosa and the color, amount, odor, and consistency of any vaginal secretions.
4. Hold two sterile cotton swabs together and swab the mucosa along the middle third of the lateral vaginal walls (Star, 1995). Two swabs are used to ensure an adequate specimen. If secretions are evident in other areas of the vagina, swab these areas as well.
5. Quickly place the two swabs in the tube of saline. Avoid touching the sides of the tube.
   It is important that the specimens be looked at within 15 minutes of collection. The specimens should not be refrigerated or stored for analysis at a later time.

■ **Pretest question #4:** The following statement is false. It is best to examine the wet-mount specimens soon after collection. However, if a delay is anticipated, refrigerate the specimen to maintain cellular integrity.

6. Determine the vaginal pH by placing a drop of vaginal secretions on pH paper (range of 3.0–5.5). Compare the color reaction with the pH reference scale to determine the vaginal pH. Do not use the swabs that you have put in the tube of saline to determine the pH. Samples for determining the pH should not be contaminated with cervical mucous or blood, as the pH of these secretions is approximately 7. Douching and recent sexual intercourse will also affect pH results.

7. After you have finished examining the patient, prepare the wet-mount slide by first gently mixing the swabs in the tube of saline.

8. Place a drop of the specimen-saline mixture on a clean glass slide by touching the dripping swabs to the slide surface. The preparation should be very "wet," so be sure there is a good-sized drop of specimen-saline mixture on the slide.

9. Place a coverslip over the specimen-saline mixture on the slide. The coverslipped area should be completely filled with the specimen mixture without excessive runoff of the mixture outside the coverslip. To avoid getting air bubbles, hold the coverslip with the thumb and forefinger perpendicular to the drop of sediment. Release the coverslip so that it falls directly on the drop of sediment. A few air bubbles is not a disaster. Just avoid looking at those areas when viewing the slide. However, many air bubbles will cause the specimen to dry out too rapidly.

10. Some clinicians prepare the saline wet mount and KOH mount on the same slide by placing the saline wet mount on one end of the slide and the KOH mount on the opposite end of the slide. Although this saves on the cost of the procedure by only using one slide for both tests, you must be very careful that the KOH solution does not leach into the saline wet-mount preparation. For this reason, it is suggested that two separate slides be used: One for the saline wet mount and one for the KOH preparation.

Examination and Interpretation of Saline Wet Mounts

The saline wet mount is examined with the low-power (10×) and high-power (40×) objectives. Be sure to close the aperture diaphragm on the condenser of the microscope when viewing wet-mount preparations.

■ **Pretest question #5:** The following statement is true. The saline wet mount is examined using both the low-power and high-power objectives.

1. Place the prepared slide in the slide holder on the microscope stage.
2. Close the aperture diaphragm on the condenser and position the low-power objective into place. For detailed instructions on how to focus the microscope see Chapter 2.
3. Scan the specimen under low power to get a general impression of the specimen. Examine at least 10 fields. One of the causes of vaginitis (ie, motile trichomonads or "clue cells") may quickly be observed, but continue to examine the specimen, as it is not unusual for a patient to have multiple infections.

■ **Pretest question #6:** The following statement is true. Multiple infections are not uncommon. Therefore be sure to examine the wet-mount specimen fully even if one cause for the vaginitis is quickly ascertained.

4. Switch to the high-power objective. As magnification is increased, it may be necessary to increase the light by opening the aperture diaphragm until optimum contrast is achieved. Again, at least 10 fields should be examined before you come to a final conclusion about the specimen.
5. Evaluate the types and number of cells present.

   A. **Epithelial cells:** Note the number and character of the epithelial cells. Report if there are sheets of epithelial cells. Normal epithelial cells have well-defined edges and look "clean" (Fig. 4-1).

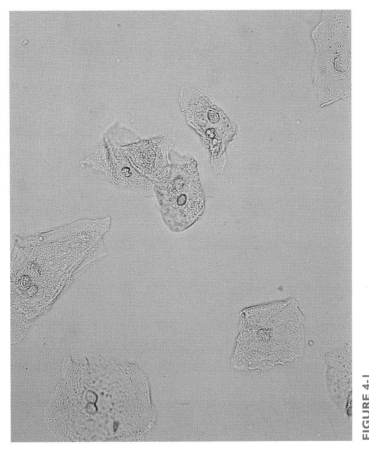

FIGURE 4-1
Normal vaginal wet mount (400×). Note clean appearance of epithelial cells.

"**Clue cells**" are epithelial cells with **many** small coc-cobacilli attached to the surface of the cell. These "clue cells" have a speckled appearance with ragged or blurred edges (Fig. 4-2).

In **cytolytic vaginosis,** the epithelial cells undergo cytoly-sis resulting in lysis of the cytoplasm of the cells, leaving disintegrating cells and naked nuclei.

B. **White blood cells** *(WBCs)*: A few WBCs (1–5 per HPF) may be a normal finding. More than 5 WBCs/HPF usually indicates vaginitis or cervicitis. The polymorphonuclear (poly, seg, PMN, neutrophil) cell is the most common WBC seen in a saline wet mount. It is 10–12 microns in size and

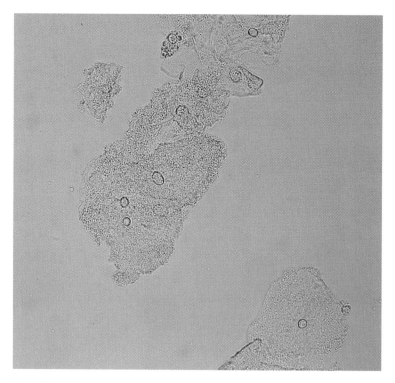

FIGURE 4-2
"Clue cells" (400×). Note speckled appearance and blurred edges of epithelial cells.

has a multisegmented nucleus and granules present in the cytoplasm. See Figures 3-5 and 3-7.

6. Evaluate the organisms present.

A. **Bacteria:** Note the number and morphology of bacteria present. Many times one can determine the presence of lactobacilli, which are large rods. These organisms are considered normal flora of the female genital tract and are thought to be important in maintaining the pH and health of the vaginal mucosa.

Recent evidence suggests that an overgrowth of lactobacilli is seen in a condition called **cytolytic vaginitis**. In this condition there is an excessive number of lactobacilli and a large number of lysed epithelial cells or naked nuclei of epithelial cells.

In patients with **bacterial vaginosis**, many small coccobacilli will be seen both on epithelial cells and in the background. See Figures 4-2 and 5-6. Note that these organisms are much smaller than the lactobacilli seen as normal flora or in cytolytic vaginitis.

Although the wet mount can be helpful in recognizing bacteria, the morphology of the bacteria can best be evaluated with a Gram stain. See Chapter 5 for instructions on how to perform a Gram stain.

B. **Candida albicans:** Look for budding yeast with pseudohyphae. Although the KOH preparation is specifically used for identifying yeast, the pseudohyphae and budding yeast cells can often be seen in the saline wet-mount preparation. If sheets of epithelial cells are present, look carefully along the edges of the epithelial cells for the protruding pseudohyphae of *C. albicans* (Fig. 4-3).

C. **Trichomonas vaginalis:** The characteristic most needed for the identification of *Trichomonas vaginalis* is motility. The organisms can vary in size (generally about the size of a WBC or larger) and shape (pear shaped, round, or triangular). Nonmotile organisms can easily be confused with WBCs or some types of epithelial cells. Therefore, it is crucial that the directional motility of these organisms be seen in order to confirm their identification. Examine clumps of WBCs carefully for motile trichomonads (Fig. 4-4; also see

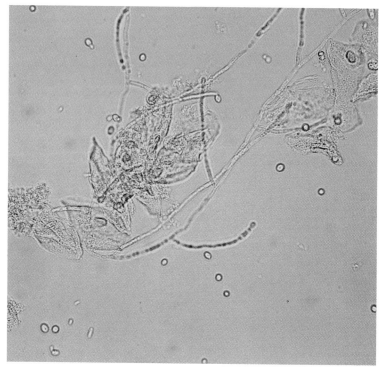

FIGURE 4-3
Yeast with pseudohyphae (400×).

Fig. 3-18). (Note: in order to show detail, Fig. 3-18 is a 1000× magnification.)

7. White blood cells may be observed with no obvious cause (that is, neither *C. albicans* nor *T. vaginalis*). Such patients need further evaluation. In patients with unexplained WBCs, consider chlamydia cervicitis, gonorrhea, Herpes simplex genitalis, or atrophic vaginitis.

Gram-staining and/or culture of appropriate specimens is necessary to diagnose these conditions. See Chapter 6 for a discussion of the proper methods of collecting and processing endocervical and urethral specimens for the diagnosis of gonorrhea and nongonococcal cervicitis/urethritis (chlamydial infections).

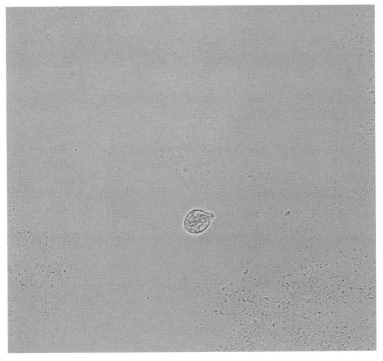

FIGURE 4-4
Trichomonas vaginalis (400×).

▐▐▐ Clinical Tips

- When you are looking at wet-mount preparations, cells or organisms may appear to jiggle continuously. This is not true motility; it is called brownian motion and is due to the constant and unequal pressure of water against the bacteria or cells. Motile organisms show a directional movement, they are going somewhere, not just vibrating back and forth. Also, placing the coverslip on the slide causes the movement of the liquid media toward the edges of the coverslip. If you see all structures moving in one direction, that is not true motility. A truly motile organism will move against the flow, or sometimes the organisms spin around in one place.
- RBCs and yeast cells have a very similar appearance. Be sure to look for buds or pseudohyphae on the yeast cells or confirm that yeast cells are present with a KOH preparation.

- Pseudohyphae can be confused with cotton fibrils or epithelial cell walls. If unsure, confirm pseudohyphae with a KOH preparation.
- Nonmotile trichomonads may resemble WBCs. In order to confirm the presence of trichomonads, they must be viable and motile, an important reason for examining wet mounts quickly after collection of the specimen.
- Other bacteria can adhere to epithelial cells and resemble "clue cells." When distinguishing clue cells be sure to look for the characteristic ragged, obscure edges.

10% POTASSIUM HYDROXIDE (KOH) PREPARATION AND EXAMINATION

The KOH preparation is a direct, microscopic test used to identify fungal elements (yeast and pseudohyphae) in vaginal secretions. This test may also be used to identify yeast and true hyphae in samples of skin scrapings, nail scrapings, and hair samples. See Chapter 7 for detailed instructions on performing KOH preparations on specimens other than vaginal secretions.

■ **Pretest question #2:** The answer is a. The KOH preparation of a vaginal discharge is used to identify **fungal elements**.

The KOH will digest or lyse epithelial cells, WBCs, RBCs, mucus, and various other cells or structures found in vaginal discharges or skin scrapings. Fungal elements (yeast, hyphae, and pseudohyphae) are not digested by the KOH and will remain clearly visible in the KOH preparation.

Preparing a Reagent

Prepare a reagent of 10% KOH solution by disolving 10 grams of KOH crystals in 90 mL of distilled water.

Procedure for Microscopic Analysis

1. Place the specimen on a clean glass slide.
2. Add 1 drop of 10% KOH. When testing vaginal secretions, before you put the coverslip on, smell the mixture. This is

the "whiff" test for bacterial vaginosis. If the specimen-KOH mixture has a fishy (amine) odor it is suggestive of bacterial vaginosis.

■ **Pretest question #1:** The answer is b. The "whiff" test is used in the diagnosis of **bacterial vaginosis**.

3. Place a coverslip over the specimen-KOH mixture on the slide. Let the slide stand for 2 to 5 minutes for clearing and digestion to occur. While you are looking at the wet-mount specimen, the KOH can be working to dissolve the cellular elements. It is usually not necessary to heat the vaginal specimen-KOH mixture.
   If the specimen is very thick or tenacious, it may be necessary to heat the specimen-KOH mixture by gently passing the slide through a flame for a few seconds. **Do not let the mixture boil.**
4. Examine the KOH mount with the low (10×) and high-dry (40×) objectives for budding yeast cells and pseudohyphae See Figure 4–3.

INTERPRETATION OF RESULTS IN THE DIAGNOSIS OF VAGINAL DISORDERS

Table 4–1 summarizes findings for vaginal discharge.

Normal Vaginal Flora

The normal vaginal discharge consists of a nonodorous, gray to white, heterogeneous, watery fluid with a pH of <4.5. The normal discharge contains epithelial cells and various microorganisms that are considered to be normal inhabitants of the vaginal tract. The most prevalent microorganisms present in the normal vagina are the lactobacilli or Döderlein bacilli. A few white blood cells may be present in normal secretions, but increased number of WBCs (>5/HPF) may indicate inflammation and should be investigated. If the vaginal wet mount and KOH fail to reveal a cause for the inflammation, then cervicitis should be suspected. Disorders of the cervix may produce a mucopurulent cervical discharge with symptoms that mimic vaginitis.

TABLE 4-1. Vaginal Discharge: Clinical and Laboratory Findings

Etiology	Discharge	WBCs	pH	Wet Mount
Normal	Scant heterogeneous, viscous to watery	Not increased (<5/HPF)	<4.5	Normal epithelial cells and lactobacilli
Candidiasis	Thick, white, cheesy	Increased (>5/HPF)	<4.5	Budding yeast with pseudohyphae
Trichomoniasis	Thin, frothy, and odorous	Increased (>5/HPF)	>4.5	Motile trichomonads
Bacterial vaginosis (BV)	Thin, milky, "fishy" odor (whiff test +)	Not increased (<5/HPF)	>4.5	"Clue cells" and lack of lactobacilli
Cytolytic vaginosis	Thick, white, cheesy	Not increased (<5/HPF)	<4.5	Lysed epithelial cells with overgrowth of lactobacilli
Atrophic vaginitis	Variable in amount, appearance, and odor	Often increased (>5/HPF)	>4.5	Immature epithelial cells, lack of lactobacilli but presence of other bacterial species.

HPF = high-power field; WBCs = white blood cells.

Neisseria gonorrhoeae and *Chlamydia trachomatis* are the most frequent causes of a purulent cervical discharge. Neither of these organisms can be seen on a wet mount or KOH preparation. Gram stain, culture, or other laboratory tests of endocervical material are necessary to diagnose these conditions. See Chapter 6 for a discussion of the proper methods of collecting and processing endocervical and urethral specimens for the diagnosis of gonorrhea and nongonococcal cervicitis/urethritis (chlamydial infections).

■ **Pretest question #3:** The answer is b. When analyzing a wet mount of a vaginal discharge, all the following cells or organisms may be observed except *N. gonorrhoeae*.

Candidiasis

Candidiasis is a relatively common infection accounting for approximately 25% of all the vaginitides (Thomason, Gelbart, & Broekhuizen, 1991). *C. albicans* is the most common yeast to cause vaginitis, although *Candida glabrata* (formerly *Torulopsis glabrata*) and *Candida tropicalis* may also cause vaginitis. Symptoms of Candidal vaginitis include pruritus, a white or yellowish discharge often described as "cottage cheese-like," erythema, and burning or soreness of the vulva. The vaginal pH of women with yeast infections is normal (<4.5).

Although the KOH preparation is used for the visualization of fungal elements, the yeast and pseudohyphae of *C. albicans* can often be seen in the saline wet mount. *C. albicans* can appear as budding yeast cells (Fig. 3-17) or as elongated cells called pseudohyphae (Fig. 4-3). The pseudohyphal form occurs only with *C. albicans* and is thought to indicate tissue invasion. Often the pseudohyphae will be found sticking out from a sheet of epithelial cells. If yeast or pseudohyphae are not found in the saline wet mount, the KOH preparation should be examined carefully for the presence of yeast and/or pseudohyphae.

Finding a few budding yeast cells in a saline wet mount or KOH preparation must be interpreted with caution. Small numbers of yeast, including *C. albicans,* may be found as normal vaginal flora in some women. More reliable than the finding of budding yeast cells is the finding of pseudohyphae. The pseudohyphal form of *C. albicans* is associated with adherence to and invasion of tissue.

Trichomoniasis

Trichomonas vaginalis is a flagellated, oval-shaped protozoan. It is a sexually transmitted parasite and accounts for approximately 15% of all cases of vaginitis (Thomason et al. 1991). Signs and symptoms of trichomoniasis include: Copious gray-white, homogenous vaginal discharge that may be malodorous, pruritus, dyspareunia, and erythema of the vaginal mucosa. The vaginal pH is >4.5.

Microscopic examination of the vaginal discharge shows many white blood cells and motile trichomonads (look very carefully within clumps of white blood cells for motile trichomonads).

Studies regarding the sensitivity of wet-mount examinations for the diagnosis of trichomonas infections vary greatly, but in clinic situations in which slides are commonly read by nonlaboratory trained personnel, the sensitivity when compared with culture is very poor (approximately 50%) (Thomason et al., 1991). Culture is available and is considered to be the "gold standard" for the diagnosis of trichomoniasis. Newer diagnostic methods such as DNA probes, enzyme-linked immunosorbent assay (ELISA), and direct fluorescent antibody (DFA) staining have recently become available and appear to have higher sensitivities than saline wet mounts.

Bacterial Vaginosis

Bacterial vaginosis (BV) is a complex polymicrobial infection involving *Gardnerella vaginalis* and anaerobic bacteria. BV accounts for approximately 30% of all the vaginitides (Thomason et al., 1991). Signs and symptoms of BV include thin, homogenous vaginal discharge, a pH of >4.5, presence of an amine or fishy odor often enhanced by the addition of KOH ("whiff" test), and vulvovaginal irritation.

Microscopic examination of the vaginal discharge shows many epithelial cells, some of which are covered with bacteria, the so-called clue cells. When distinguishing clue cells from normal epithelial cells it is important to look at the edges of the cell. A clue cell by definition has jagged, or blurred edges. Lactobacilli are reduced or absent and there is no inflammatory response; thus, there is no increase in WBCs. If clue cells are present with an increased number of WBCs, then a second infectious agent should be sought to account for the inflammatory response.

Cytolytic Vaginosis

Cytolytic vaginosis, also known as lactobacilli overgrowth syndrome, is a condition characterized by increased exfoliation of the squamous epithelium of the vagina. Signs and symptoms include nonodorous, thick, white discharge, burning, and dyspareunia. (**Note:** Visual examination of the discharge may lead the clinician to make an inaccurate diagnosis of infection with *C. albicans.*) This condition is thought to be caused by an overgrowth of lactobacilli, which results in increased acid production and lysis of epithelial cell cytoplasm.

The saline wet mount will show an increase in the numbers of epithelial cells with cellular debris from lysed epithelial cells, naked nuclei of lysed epithelial cells, copious number of large rods, and no increase in WBCs.

Atrophic Vaginitis

Estrogen deficiency, as seen in postmenopausal women, may cause a thinning of the vaginal mucosa and a decrease in glycogen in the vaginal epithelium. This decrease in glycogen results in a reduction in lactic acid production with a corresponding increase in vaginal pH and change in microflora (lactobacilli replaced by gastrointestinal tract organisms). The majority of women with an atrophic vagina are asymptomatic, but occasionally inflammation occurs and patients may complain of vaginal soreness, burning, and discharge often precipitated by intercourse.

The saline wet mount frequently shows an increase in white blood cells in association with small, immature squamous epithelial cells. Lactobacilli are replaced by mixed gastrointestinal tract organisms, mostly gram-negative rods.

CHAPTER 4 PRETEST ANSWERS

1. The answer is b, bacterial vaginosis. The "whiff" test is used in the diagnosis of bacterial vaginosis. When KOH is added to the vaginal discharge of a patient with bacterial vaginosis, an amine or "fishy" odor is released. This is a positive "whiff" test and is suggestive of bacterial vaginosis.

2. The answer is a, fungal elements. The KOH preparation is used to identify fungal elements. A 10% solution of potassium hydroxide (KOH) will dissolve cells, but not fungi. This makes visualization of yeast, pseudohyphae and true hyphae easier.

3. The answer is b, *N. gonorrhoeae*. In order to see *Neisseria gonorrhoeae*, a Gram stain or methylene blue stain must be done. It cannot be seen on a saline wet mount.

4. False. *T. vaginalis* is very sensitive to changes in temperature and therefore specimens should not be refrigerated. The speciman should be examined within 15 minutes of collection.

5. True

6. True

CHAPTER 4 POSTTEST

1. Describe the function of the potassium hydroxide reagent in the KOH mount.

2. Yeast cells can often resemble RBCs when viewed microscopically in a saline wet mount. What are two microscopic characteristics of yeast that differentiate them from RBCs?

3. What feature of *Trichomonas vaginalis* is most important in its identification?

4. Describe the appearance of a "clue cell." What feature of the cell is most important in identifying it as a clue cell.

5. What is the identification of the organisms and cells seen in Figure 4-5?

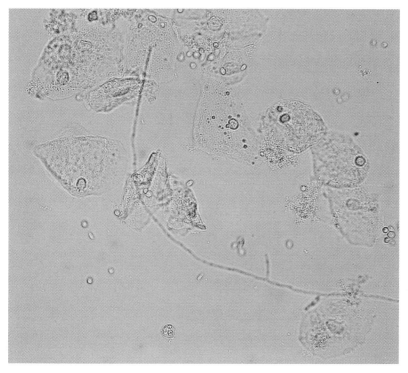

FIGURE 4-5
Posttest question #5 (400×).

CHAPTER 4 POSTTEST ANSWERS

1. The potassium hydroxide (KOH) dissolves cells and mucus but does not dissolve fungi. The KOH preparation is used to identify fungal elements (yeast, pseudohyphae, and hyphae) in vaginal secretions, skin scrapings, and hair specimens.

2. Budding and pseudohyphae

3. In order to identify *T. vaginalis,* the organism must be motile.

4. A "clue cell" is a squamous epithelial cell that has been covered with many small coccobacillary bacteria. The feature most important in the identification of a clue cell is a ragged, blurred border on the cell.

5. Yeast with pseudohyphae and epithelial cells

REFERENCES

Star, W. (1995). Vaginitis. In W. L. Star, L. Lommel, & M.T. Shannon (Eds.), *Women's primary care: Protocols for practice* (pp. 12–197). Washington, D.C.: American Nurses' Association.

Thomason, J. L., Gelbart, S. M., & Broekhuizen, F. F. (1991). Office and clinical laboratory diagnosis of vulvovaginal infections: An overview. In B. Horowitz and P. Mardh (Eds.), *Vaginitis and vaginosis* (pp. 93–108). New York: Wiley-Liss.

SUGGESTED READINGS

Baron, E. J., Cassell, G. H., Duffy, L. B., Eschenbach, D. A., Greenwook, J. R., Harvey, S. M., Madinger, N. E., Peterson, E. M., & Waites, K. B. (1993). Laboratory diagnosis of female genital tract infections, *Cumitech 17A.* Washington, DC: American Society for Microbiology.

Eschenbach, D. (1993). *Bacterial vaginosis: An overview.* Elk Grove Village, IL: Curatek Pharmaceuticals.

Horowitz, B. J. & Mardh, P. A. (Eds.) (1991). *Vaginitis and vaginosis.* New York: Wiley-Liss.

Pasteorek II, J. G. (1994). *Obstetric and gynecologic infectious disease.* New York: Raven Press.

Reife, C. M. (1995). Office gynecology for the primary care physician, part I: Vaginitis, the Papanicolaou smear, contraception, and post-menopausal estrogen replacement. *Medical Clinics of North America.* *80*, 299–303.

Sobel, J. D. (1992). Vulvovaginitis. *Dermatologic Clinics. 10*, 339–359.

Sweet. R. L. & Gibbs, R. S. (1995). *Infectious diseases of the female genital tract.* Baltimore: Williams and Wilkins.

Gram Staining

The Gram stain is one of the most important tools in clinical microbiology. It separates most bacteria into two groups: gram-positive bacteria, which stain purple, and gram-negative bacteria, which stain pink to red. (Bacteria stain differently because of differences in the structures and chemical compositions of their cell walls.) In addition to determining gram reaction, the shape and arrangement of bacteria may also be determined with the Gram stain (Box 5-1).

OBJECTIVES

Upon completion of this chapter, the reader will be able to:

1. Prepare slides from various clinical specimens (urine, sputum, urethral discharge, endocervical and vaginal discharge) for Gram staining.
2. Perform a Gram stain properly.
3. Examine Gram-stained smears microscopically and identify the following:
   - Gram-positive cocci in pairs (diplococci), chains, or clusters
   - Gram-negative diplococci
   - Gram-negative rods
   - Gram-positive rods
   - Yeast and pseudohyphae
   - Epithelial cells
   - Polymorphonuclear cells (also known as polys)
4. Discuss the clinical relevance of microscopic findings on Gram-stained smears of urethral, endocervical, vaginal, sputum, and urine specimens.

Box 5-1. The Shape and Arrangement of Bacteria

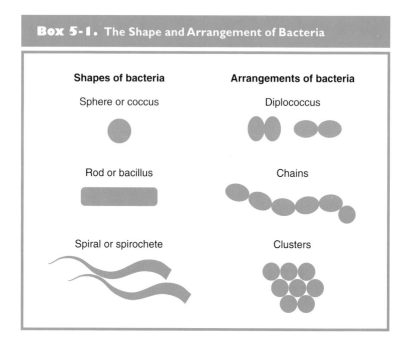

OBJECTIVES (Continued)

Please take the pretest. After completion of the pretest, read the material in the chapter.

Chapter 5 Pretest

Questions 1–5: Answer true or false.

1. Gram-positive organisms retain the primary dye and therefore appear purple at the end of the Gram-stain procedure.

2. When preparing slides to be Gram stained, the specimen is placed on a clean glass slide and then gently heated over a flame to dry the material on the slide before it is stained.

3. In a properly performed Gram stain, human cells, such as polymorphonuclear cells, should be gram positive.

4. The decolorization step of the Gram stain should be done for exactly 15 seconds.

5. Gram stains of urine specimens should be done on unspun urine specimens.

6. Name the three basic shapes of bacteria.

Questions 7–9: State the Gram reaction and morphology of the following organisms:

7. *Neisseria gonorrhoeae*

8. *Streptococcus pneumoniae*

9. Lactobacilli

The pretest answers will appear throughout the text of the chapter and before the posttest.

SLIDE PREPARATION

1. Material to be stained is dropped (if liquid) or rolled (if present on a swab) onto the surface of a clean, dry glass slide. Smears should not be too thick, as thick smears are hard to stain properly.
2. The smear is then allowed to **air dry**. It is important that slides be totally dry before continuing with the staining procedure. To speed the drying process, smears may be placed on a slide warmer at 60°C or put in a 37°C incubator. The slides should not be passed through a flame to dry. Heat fixing should be done only after the slide is completely dry.

■ **Pretest question #2:** The following statement is false. When preparing slides to be Gram stained, the specimen is placed on a clean glass slide and then gently heated over a flame to dry the material on the slide before it is stained.

3. After the slide is dry, it is fixed so that the material remains on the slide during the staining procedure. One common method of fixation is gentle heating of the slide. Hold the slide in your hand and quickly pass it through a flame (specimen side up and away from the flame). Then touch the slide to the back of your hand. The slide should be warm, but not hot. Repeat three or four times. **DO NOT OVERHEAT**—temperature should be just tolerable to skin on the back of the hand. Heat fixing is a gentle process and the slide should never get hot. If you burn your hand, you have also burned the specimen.

    An alternative method for fixing the specimen to the glass slide is methanol fixation. Slides that have air dried are flooded with 95% methanol for 1 minute. The methanol is then drained off and the slides are again dried before staining. Although more costly and time consuming, this is the preferred method of fixation. It preserves cellular morphology (often cells become distorted or lysed when heat fixed) and eliminates the possibility of overheating the slide.

GRAM STAIN PROCEDURE

After the slide is heat fixed, it must cool before you begin the staining procedure. If the slide is stained before it is allowed to cool, the crystal violet will precipitate on the slide, making interpretation difficult. If the slide is methanol fixed, it should be allowed to dry before staining to ensure adequate fixation.

The reagents used in the Gram stain are:

- Crystal violet—primary stain. Stains all material purple.
- Gram's iodine—mordant. This reagent fixes the crystal violet to bacteria having a certain cell wall composition (gram-positive organisms).
- Acetone/alcohol mixture—decolorizer. This reagent removes the primary stain (crystal violet) from all bacteria and cells that do not have the cell wall composition of gram-positive organisms.
- Basic fuchsin or safranin—counterstain. This reagent stains all bacteria and cells that have been decolorized with the acetone/alcohol reagent.

The steps of the staining procedure are as follows:

1. Cover the heat- or methanol-fixed smear with crystal violet and allow the stain to remain on the slide for 5–10 seconds (timing of this step is not critical); wash off with tap water; drain water.
2. Cover the smear with Gram's iodine and allow the reagent to remain on the slide for 5–10 seconds (timing of this step is not critical). Wash the slide off with tap water; drain the water.
3. TIMING IS CRITICAL. Holding the slide at about a 45° angle, run the decolorizing agent (acetone/alcohol) over the slide and watch the excess run off the bottom edge of the slide. Continue decolorizing until the purple dye no longer runs off the slide with the decolorizer (ie, the excess dripping off the bottom edge of the slide is colorless, no purple color is present). Immediately wash with tap water; drain the water.

■ **Pretest question #4:** The following statement is false. The decolorization step of the Gram stain should be done for exactly 15 seconds.

In clinical specimens, the best criterion for adequate de-colorization is that the nuclei of the polymorphonuclear or epithelial cells should be stained gram-negative (pink). If the nuclear material is purple, the slide may not have been decolorized adequately. (See Fig. 5-2.)

4. Cover the smear with basic fuchsin (or safranin) and allow to stand for 5–10 seconds (timing of this step is not critical). Wash the slide off with tap water; drain the water.

5. Blot dry and examine microscopically. See Chapter 2 for detailed instructions on how to microscopically examine a Gram-stained smear.

The microscopic appearance after each step of the Gram stain is indicated in Table 5-1.

INTERPRETATION OF GRAM STAINS

Interpretation of a Gram-stained smear requires determination of the color, shape, and arrangement of any bacteria that may be present as well as the type of cells present in the specimen.

When looking at a Gram-stained smear, you should look in a relatively thin area of the slide. If the specimen is very thick or tenacious, it may be hard to decolorize the thicker areas of the slide. Figures 5-1 and 5-2 are views of different areas of the same slide. Note that in Figure 5-1 the nuclei of the polymorphonuclear cells are pink and the organisms are stained gram-positive. The polymorphonuclear cells are relatively spread out and the background is light pink. Figure 5-2 shows a very thick area of the

TABLE 5-1. Appearance of Bacteria After Each Step of the Gram Stain

	Microscopic Appearance	
	Gram positive	*Gram negative*
Crystal violet	Purple	Purple
Gram's iodine	Purple	Purple
Acetone-alcohol	Purple	Colorless
Basic fuchsin or safranin	Purple	Pink to red

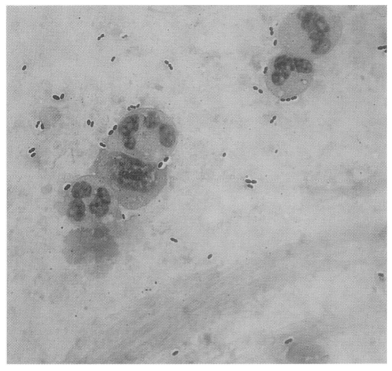

FIGURE 5-1
Properly done Gram stain. Note gram-positive bacteria and gram-negative cells (1,000×)

same slide. The nuclei of the polymorphonuclear cells are gram positive and the background is very dark. When looking at Gram stains, one should not look in these very thick areas of the slide.

Color or Gram Reaction of Organisms

- Gram positive organisms retain the crystal violet and therefore appear **purple** after Gram staining.

Pretest question #1: The following statement is true. Gram-positive organisms retain the primary dye and therefore appear purple at the end of the Gram stain procedure.

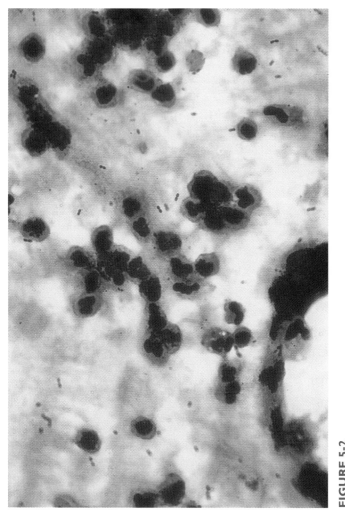

FIGURE 5-2
Improperly done Gram stain. Note partially gram-positive cells (1,000×).

- Gram-negative organisms are decolorized with the acetone/alcohol reagent and are therefore stained with the counterstain (basic fuchsin or safranin) and appear **pink to red** after staining.

Shape of Organisms

- Cocci: Round or slightly oval organisms
- Rods or bacilli: Rod-shaped organisms. They may be long or short, fat or thin, and some may appear curved.
- Spirochetes: Spiral-shaped bacteria. Most spirochetes do not stain with the Gram stain and therefore will not be visible with this staining procedure.

Pretest question #6: The three basic shapes of bacteria are rods, cocci, and spirochetes.

Arrangement of Organisms

- Clusters: See Figure 5-12.
- Chains: Three or more organisms attached end to end. See Figure 5-14.
- Diplococci: Two cocci paired together. See Figures 5-3 and 5-9B.

Cells Commonly Seen on Gram-Stained Smears of Clinical Specimens

- Epithelial cells: Large cell with small nucleus. See Figures 5-5 and 5-8 A and B.
- White blood cells (WBCs): The WBCs most commonly seen are polymorphonuclear cells. They are much smaller than epithelial cells and have multiple segments to their nucleus. Many times polymorphonuclear cells will be broken apart when doing the Gram stain and will be difficult to identify. See Figures 5-3 and 5-9A and B.
- Mononuclear cells: Macrophages or histiocytes are sometimes seen in Gram-stained smears. They are larger than polymorphonuclear cells and do not have segmented nuclei.

All cellular material should stain gram-negative. If the cells are gram-positive the smear may not have been decolorized long enough. Such a smear will be difficult to interpret.

■ **Pretest question #3:** The following statement is false. In a properly performed Gram stain, human cells, such as polymorphonuclear cells, should be gram-positive.

SPECIMENS COMMONLY EXAMINED WITH THE GRAM STAIN

The Gram stain is used on many specimens; only a few of these are done in the office laboratory, however. The most commonly examined specimens will be discussed below. Specimen collection will not be covered in this chapter.

Urethral Discharge

Urethral specimens are examined to diagnose gonococcal urethritis and nongonococcal urethritis. See Chapter 6 for instructions on how to collect urethral specimens.

Slide Preparation

Specimens are generally collected on calcium alginate or Dacron swabs. Roll the swab gently across a small section of the slide. The swab should be rolled across the slide, rather than streaked, to better preserve cellular morphology and to ensure that all areas of the swab come in contact with the slide. (Because specimens may need to be cultured for *N. gonorrhoeae*, two swabs should be collected; one should be used for culture and the other for Gram stain. Swabs that have been rolled on a slide should not be used for culture.) Allow slide to air dry, then heat- or methanol-fix the slide and proceed with the Gram-staining procedure.

Interpretation of Results
- Finding polymorphonuclear cells in urethral specimens indicates urethritis.
- Finding gram-negative diplococci within the polymorphonuclear cells (intracellular) is strong evidence for the diagnosis of gonorrhea (Fig. 5-3). Gonorrhea is caused by the organ-

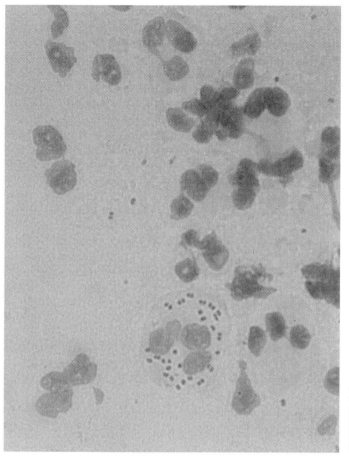

FIGURE 5-3
Gram stain of urethral discharge. Note gram-negative intracellular diplococci (1,000×).

ism *Neisseria gonorrhoeae*, which is a gram-negative diplococci often found within polymorphonuclear cells. Smear-positive urethral specimens need not be confirmed with culture for *N. gonorrhoeae*.

■ **Pretest question #7:** *N. gonorrhoeae* is a gram-negative diplococci.

* Finding polymorphonuclear cells with no intracellular gram-negative diplococci is suggestive of nongonococcal urethritis. Specimens without gram-negative intracellular diplococci should be cultured to rule out gonorrhea definitively. The organism most commonly causing nongonococcal urethritis is *Chlamydia trachomatis*. This organism cannot be seen on Gram stain.

▓▓▓▓ **Clinical Tip**

* Although Gram staining is the method of choice for microscopically looking at urethral smears, some practitioners use the more simple methylene blue stain on urethral smears from males.

Methylene Blue Procedure

Prepare the slide as for Gram stain. Air dry, and heat- or methanol-fix the prepared slide. Cover the slide with methylene blue for 1 minute. Wash with water and blot dry. Examine with the oil-immersion (100×) lens.

Interpretation of Results

With this stain, all cells and structures stain blue. If characteristic diplococci are seen within polymorphonuclear cells, then a diagnosis of gonorrhea can be made (Fig. 5-4). If many polymorphonuclear cells are seen with no characteristic diplococci, then nongonococcal urethritis is likely. However, a culture for *N. gonorrhoeae* should be done to rule out gonorrhea definitively.

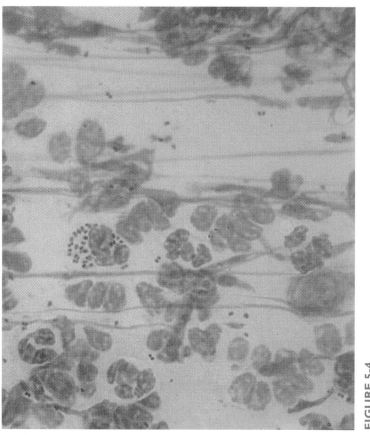

FIGURE 5-4
Methylene blue stain of urethral discharge. Note intracellular diplococci (1,000×).

Endocervical Discharge

A Gram stain of endocervical discharge can be helpful in determining the causative agent in a case of cervicitis but is not as sensitive or specific as a Gram stain of urethral discharge. There is a significant number of culture-positive cases of gonorrhea in women in which gram-negative diplococci were not seen on the Gram stain. Conversely, because the female genital tract has such a diverse normal flora, some organisms that normally reside in the female genital tract can be mistaken for gram-negative diplococci. Thus, false positive results also occur. Because of these problems, many practitioners have ceased doing Gram stains on endocervical specimens. Culturing or other methods for the identification of *N. gonorrhoeae* or *C. trachomatis* must be done in order to determine the cause of cervicitis. See Chapter 6 for a more detailed discussion on diagnosis of cervicitis.

If a Gram stain is done on an endocervical discharge, the specimen swab should be processed in the same manner as a urethral discharge swab. Methylene blue stains should not be done on endocervical specimens.

Vaginal Discharge

Saline wet mounts and KOH preparations are the microscopic techniques most commonly employed when examining vaginal discharge specimens. However, Gram stains of vaginal secretions can aid in the diagnosis of various clinical conditions.

Slide Preparation

Specimens are generally collected on sterile cotton swabs (see Chapter 4). Roll the swab gently across a small section of the slide. Allow the slide to air dry, heat- or methanol-fix, and then proceed with the Gram-staining procedure.

Interpretation of Results

- Normal vaginal smear: Squamous epithelial cells (the cells should stain gram-negative; if they appear gram positive you did not decolorize sufficiently) and large gram-positive bacilli (lactobacilli). You may also see a few WBCs and RBCs (Fig. 5–5).

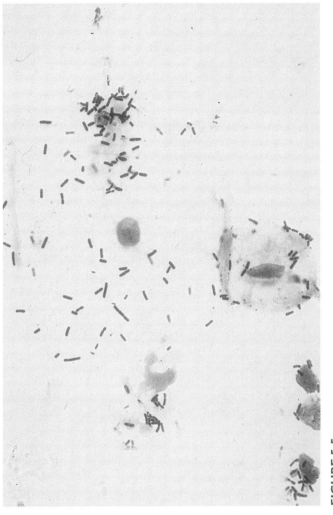

FIGURE 5-5

Gram stain of normal vaginal smear. Note large gram-positive rods (lactobacilli) (1,000×).

■ **Pretest question #9:** Lactobacilli are gram-positive rods.

- Bacterial vaginosis (BV): Many epithelial cells, some covered with gram-variable coccobacilli ("clue cells"). The background will also contain numerous bacteria, both gram negative and gram positive. There will be a noticeable absence of lactobacilli (Fig. 5-6). WBCs are absent or rare in women with BV; mixed infections are common, however. The presence of both clue cells and increased WBCs indicates a coexisting infection (eg, trichomonas, yeast, gonorrhea, or chlamydia).
- Candida vaginitis: Many squamous epithelial cells, gram-positive budding yeast with pseudohyphae. Many times the yeast will be associated with a sheet of epithelial cells. WBCs and lactobacilli may also be present (Fig. 5-7).

Sputum

Sputum specimens are examined from patients with signs and symptoms of pneumonia in hopes of detecting a bacterial cause. It is important that sputum, and not saliva, be tested for both the Gram stain and culture. If the specimen is watery and foamy, then it is most likely saliva and not sputum. Sputum is thick and tenacious and many times will be streaked with yellowish or greenish flecks. These flecks are often WBCs and are the material that should be obtained for Gram stain.

Slide Preparation

Pick up any purulent material that may be present in the specimen on a sterile swab. Gently rotate the swab on a clean glass slide. Be sure the slide is not too thick. You should be able to see through the material on the slide. It should not be very opaque. Allow slide to air dry, heat- or methanol-fix, and then proceed with the Gram-staining procedure.

Interpretation of Results

Examine the slide under low power (10×). Scan several fields to determine whether the specimen is acceptable. An acceptable specimen should contain polymorphonuclear cells and have fewer

(text continues on page 135)

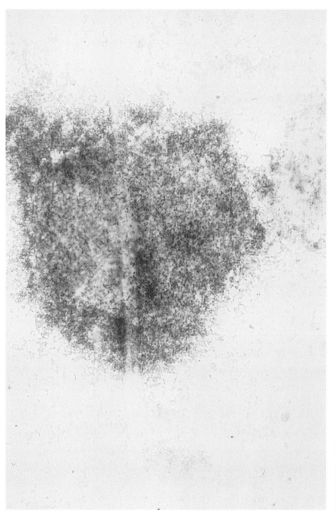

FIGURE 5-6

Gram stain of "clue cell." Note large numbers of small gram-positive and gram-negative bacteria, many of which are attached to epithelial cells (1,000×).

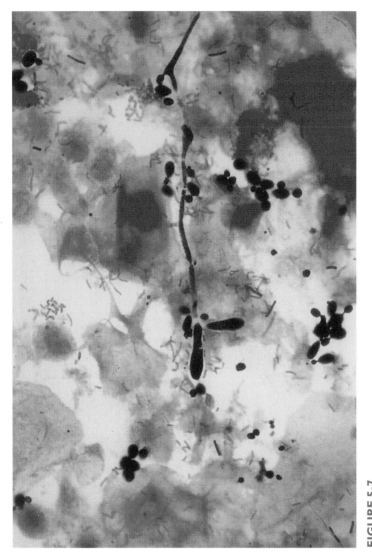

FIGURE 5-7
Epithelial cells and budding yeast with pseudohyphae (1,000×).

than 10 epithelial cells per low-power field (LPF). If there are more than 10 epithelial cells per LPF, then the specimen is most likely saliva and should not be used for diagnosis. If the specimen is unacceptable, collect another sample (Figs. 5-8 and 5-9).

If the specimen is acceptable, find a relatively thin area of the slide that has a number of polymorphonuclear cells. Place a drop of oil on the slide and rotate the oil-immersion (100×) lens into place. Examine several areas of the slide under oil immersion to determine whether there is a predominating organism present on the slide. Look especially in areas where there are many polymorphonuclear cells.

The following organisms are common causes of pneumonia:

- *Streptococcus pneumoniae:* Gram-positive diplococci. See Figure 5-9B.
- *Haemophilus influenzae:* Tiny gram-negative rod; may appear coccoid and is often called a coccobacilli (Fig. 5-10).
- *Klebsiella pneumoniae:* Large gram-negative rods (Fig. 5-11).
- *Staphylococcus aureus:* Gram-positive cocci in clusters (Fig. 5-12).
- Viruses: Not seen on Gram stain
- *Mycoplasma pneumoniae*: Not seen on Gram stain.

■ **Pretest answer #8:** *Streptococcus pneumoniae* is a gram-positive diplococci.

Urine

A urine Gram stain can be very useful in the diagnosis and treatment of urinary tract infections. Finding one or more bacteria per oil-immersion field in a drop of **unspun** urine correlates well with a colony count of more than 100,000 organisms per millileter of urine. Finding more than 100,000 organisms per millileter has traditionally been considered the cutoff point for significant bacteriuria. Recent studies have shown, however, that colony counts as low as 100 organisms per mL may be significant if the patient is symptomatic. For this reason, culture should be considered when a urinary tract infection is suspected, either because of symptoms or results of a routine urinalysis.

(text continues on page 141)

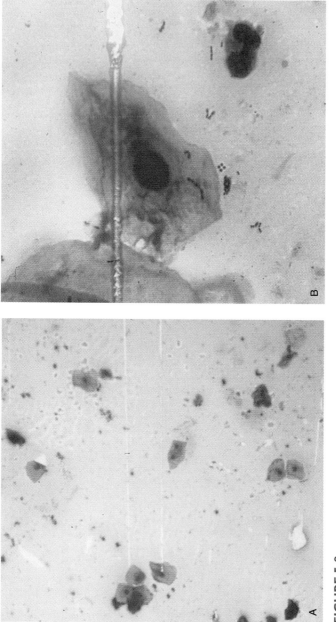

FIGURE 5-8
(A) Low power (100×). (B) Oil immersion (1,000×). Unacceptable sputum specimen. Note large numbers of epithelial cells and variety of organisms.

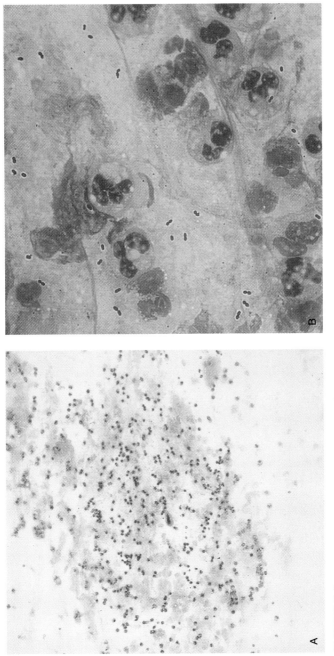

FIGURE 5-9

(A) Low power (100×). (B) Oil immersion (1000×). Acceptable sputum specimen. Note large numbers of polymorphonuclear cells and one predominate organism. Gram-positive diplococci (*Streptococcus pneumoniae*).

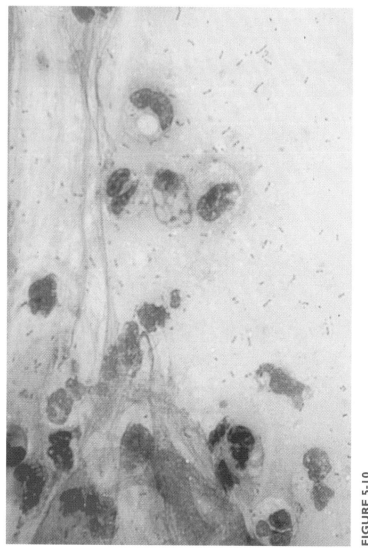

FIGURE 5-10
Sputum with tiny gram-negative coccobacilli (*Haemophilus influenzae*) (1,000×).

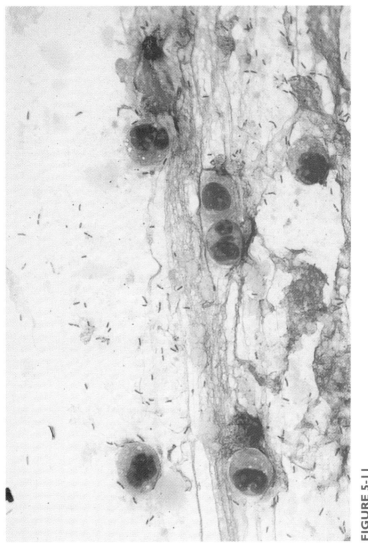

FIGURE 5-11
Sputum with large gram-negative rods. (*Klebsiella pneumoniae*) (1,000×).

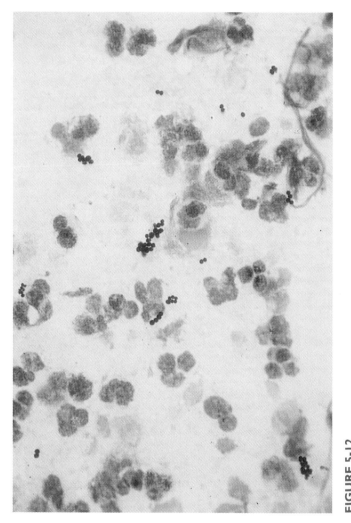

FIGURE 5-12
Sputum with gram-positive cocci in clusters (*Staphylococcus aureus*) (1,000×).

■ **Pretest question #5:** The following statement is true. Gram stains of urine specimens should be done on unspun urine specimens.

Slide Preparation

Place a drop of urine on a clean microscope slide. Allow slide to air dry, heat- or methanol-fix, and then proceed with the Gram-staining procedure.

Interpretation of Results

Seeing one or more organisms per oil-immersion field indicates significant bacteriuria (colony count higher than 100,000 organisms per milliliter). Gram-negative rods are the most frequently seen organisms causing urinary tract infections. However, gram-positive cocci may also be seen (Figs. 5-13 and 5-14).

The presence of two or more different bacterial types, or a significant number of epithelial cells suggests contamination and the need for collecting another specimen.

QUALITY CONTROL AND SAFETY

A control slide containing known gram-negative and gram-positive organisms should be used to control your reagents and techniques. How often the controls should be run depends on the number of Gram stains performed. For example, if many Gram stains are done, quality control should be done daily. If Gram stains are only infrequently done (fewer than one per day), then a control slide should be done with each Gram stain.

Control slides may be purchased from laboratory supply companies or made in-house by using cultures of known gram-positive and gram-negative organisms.

Gram-staining may not kill all organisms on a slide. Therefore, Gram-stained slides should be handled as other infectious material.

(text continues on page 144)

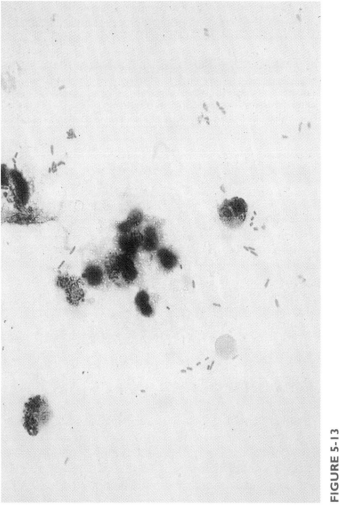

FIGURE 5-13
Urine with polys and gram-negative rods (*Escherichia coli*) (1,000×).

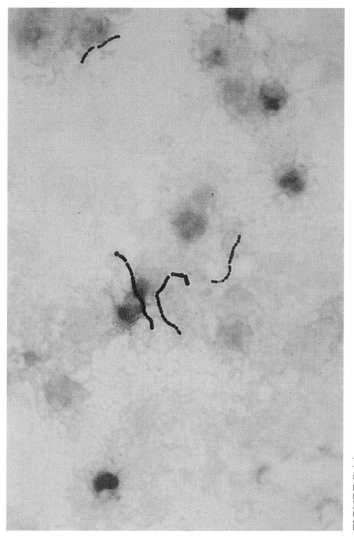

FIGURE 5-14
Urine with polymorphonuclear cells and gram-positive cocci in chains (*Enterococcus* or *Streptococcus*) (1,000×).

CHAPTER 5 PRETEST ANSWERS

1. True

2. False. The specimen should be allowed to air dry on the slide before it is heated.

3. False. Cells should appear gram negative. If they are gram positive, it indicates that the slide may not have been decolorized long enough.

4. False. Timing of the decolorization step is critical; however, no one time will be right for all slides. How long you decolorize depends on the thickness of the smear and the consistency of the specimen. Thick, tenacious specimens such as sputum require longer decolorization than thinner specimens such as urine. Review the Gram-stain procedure for detailed instructions on how to decolorize your slide.

5. True

6. The three basic shapes of bacteria are rods or bacilli, cocci, and spirochetes.

7. *N. gonorrhoeae* is a gram-negative diplococci.

8. *S. pneumoniae* is a gram-positive diplococci.

9. Lactobacilli are large gram-positive rods.

CHAPTER 5 POSTTEST

1. List the Gram-stain reagents in the order that they are used.

Questions 2–4: You have done a Gram stain on a vaginal discharge. If the staining has been done correctly, the following will be observed microscopically. Fill in the blanks with the appropriate color.

2. Gram-positive organisms will appear _____.

3. Gram-negative organisms will appear _____.

4. Epithelial cells and WBCs will appear _____.

5. Describe the procedure you would use to prepare a slide of a urine specimen for Gram staining.

Question 6: Multiple choice. Select the one best answer.

6. In the Gram-stain procedure, bacteria on a slide are exposed to an acetone/alcohol mixture. The purpose of this step is

   a. to adhere the cells to the slide.

   b. to retain the pink dye within all bacteria.

   c. to remove the purple dye from gram-negative bacteria.

   d. to facilitate the entry of the blue dye into the gram-negative bacteria.

7. Describe the criteria used to determine whether a sputum sample is acceptable for Gram stain and culture.

8. The finding of gram-negative diplococci within polymorphonuclear cells in a urethral discharge is diagnostic of what disease?

CHAPTER 5 POSTTEST ANSWERS

1. The reagents used in the Gram stain, in order of use, are:
   Crystal violet
   Gram's iodine
   Acetone/alcohol
   Safranin or basic fuchsin.

2. Gram-positive organisms are purple.

3. Gram-negative organisms are pink to red.

4. Epithelial cells and WBCs are pink to red.

5. A drop of unspun urine is placed on a clean glass slide and allowed to air dry. After the slide is dry, it is gently heat or methanol fixed. When the slide has cooled to room temperature (if heat fixed) or dried (if methanol fixed) it is ready for Gram staining.

6. The correct answer is c. The acetone/alcohol is a decolorizing agent. It removes the primary dye (crystal violet) from gram-negative bacteria.

7. An acceptable sputum sample should have fewer than 10 epithelial cells per LPF. If the specimen contains more than 10 epithelial cells per LPF, it is most likely contaminated with saliva. Also, the specimen should have polymorphonuclear cells and one predominating organism. If many different types of organisms are present, it also suggests that the specimen is contaminated with saliva.

8. Gonorrhea is diagnosed by finding gram-negative diplococci within polymorphonuclear cells in a urethral exudate.

SUGGESTED READINGS

Baron, E. J., Peterson, L. R., & Finegold, S. M. (Eds.). (1994). *Diagnostic microbiology* (9th ed.). St. Louis: Mosby.

Murray, P. R., Baron, E. J., Pfaller, M. A., Tenover, F. C., & Yolken, R. H. (Eds.). (1995). *Manual of clinical microbiology* (6th ed.). Washington, DC: American Society for Microbiology.

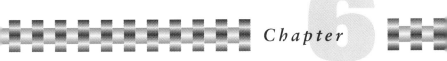

Collection and Handling of Endocervical and Urethral Specimens

Cervicitis and urethritis are common conditions affecting millions of individuals each year. The infectious agents that cause cervicitis/urethritis are generally sexually transmitted and can be divided into gonococcal (GC) cervicitis/urethritis and nongonococcal cervicitis/urethritis (NGC, NGU). GC is caused by the organism *Neisseria gonorrhoeae*. NGC/NGU may be caused by several different organisms; however, *Chlamydia trachomatis* is the organism most clearly associated with NGC/NGU.

Clinically there is much overlap between GC and NGC/NGU, and a differential diagnosis should not be made solely on clinical grounds. In order to diagnose the etiology of cervicitis/urethritis, laboratory testing must be done. The sensitivity and specificity of laboratory tests for the diagnosis of cervicitis/urethritis are dependent upon the quality of the specimen obtained for analysis. Strict adherence to the steps for collecting and handling endocervical and urethral specimens will increase both the sensitivity and specificity of diagnostic laboratory testing.

OBJECTIVES

Upon completion of this chapter, the reader will be able to:

1. Describe the two most common causes of urethritis and cervicitis.

OBJECTIVES (Continued)

2. Describe the laboratory tests used in the diagnosis of urethritis and cervicitis.
3. Describe the proper techniques for the collection and handling of urethral and endocervical specimens.
4. Correlate laboratory and clinical findings to diagnose the causes of urethritis and cervicitis.

Please take the pretest. After completion of the pretest, read the material in the chapter.

CHAPTER 6 PRETEST

Questions 1–5: Answer true or false.

1. A Gram stain of an endocervical discharge specimen is a reliable method for diagnosing cervicitis caused by *N. gonorrhoeae*.

2. The vaginal speculum used for visualizing the vagina and cervix should be moistened with a water-soluble gel to avoid any interference with specimen collection.

3. Sterile Dacron swabs should be used for collecting endocervical specimens for microbiological culture of both *N. gonorrhoeae* and *C. trachomatis*.

4. Urethral specimens for microbiological cultures should be obtained immediately after the individual has voided.

5. Collection of specimens for culture of *N. gonorrhoeae* should be obtained prior to specimens for culture of *C. trachomatis*.

Question 6: *Multiple choice. Select the one best answer.*

6. Which one of the following findings would be **most** consistent with a diagnosis of mucopurulent cervicitis?

    a. Discharge with 1–3 red blood cells per high-power field (HPF).

    b. Discharge with more than 10 WBCs per HPF.

    c. Discharge with more than five epithelial cells per HPF.

    d. Discharge with a "fishy" or amine odor.

7. Describe the procedure for handling an inoculated Thayer-Martin plate.

8. Describe the procedure for handling a specimen collected for tissue culture of *C. trachomatis* if there is a delay in transporting the specimen to the laboratory.

The pretest answers will appear throughout the text of the chapter and before the posttest.

ENDOCERVICAL SPECIMENS

Mucopurulent cervicitis (MPC) is a common condition among young, sexually active women. The clinical criteria for the diagnosis of MPC are the presence of a mucopurulent discharge from the endocervix and erythema, edema, and friability of the cervix. It is generally accepted that finding more than 10 WBCs per HPF on the microscopic examination of the cervical discharge is indicative of MPC.

■ **Pretest question #6:** The answer is b. The finding most consistent with a diagnosis of MPC is a discharge with more than 10 WBCs per HPF.

The two most common bacterial causes of MPC are *N. gonorrhoeae* and *C. trachomatis*. Microbiological culture is the "gold standard" for the diagnosis of both of these infections. These organisms, however, are different in their pathology and growth requirements and therefore specimen collection, handling, and culture methods are specific for each organism. Dual infections with both organisms are prevalent, and it is generally recommended to do testing for both *N. gonorrhoeae* and *C. trachomatis*.

When culturing for both *N. gonorrhoeae* and *C. trachomatis*, separate specimens should be collected. The swab for *N. gonorrhoeae* should be collected first, as this organism is present in the urethral discharge or exudate. *C. trachomatis* is an obligate intracellular organism found in columnar or cuboidal epithelial cells. Isolation of the organism is dependent upon removal of any urethral exudate so as to obtain epithelial cells.

Newer tests such as direct fluorescent antibody (DFA), enzyme immunoassay (EIA), DNA probes, and polymerase chain reaction (PCR) are increasing in sensitivity and specificity, and many laboratories are replacing culture with these faster and more convenient testing methods. Each of these methodologies will have specific specimen collection materials and information on the proper specimen collection and handling to be used for the test employed. Be sure to be familiar with the testing procedure used in your laboratory. Use the collection and handling materials and techniques appropriate for the test method that is in use.

Specimen Collection for Culture of *Neisseria gonorrhoeae*

In women, the endocervical mucosa is the site most commonly infected with *N. gonorrhoeae*, and endocervical specimens should be obtained for diagnosis of GC. Diagnosis of endocervical infections with *N. gonorrhoeae* generally requires the isolation and identification of the organism by culture. Unlike urethral specimens, Gram stains of direct smears from endocervical specimens lack specificity and sensitivity. Therefore, Gram stains of endocervical specimens for the diagnosis of infection with *N. gonorrhoeae* must be interpreted with caution. Methylene blue stains, which are commonly done on urethral specimens (see Chapter 5), should not be done on endocervical specimens.

■ **Pretest question #1:** The following statement is false. A Gram stain of an endocervical discharge specimen is a reliable method for diagnosing cervicitis caused by *N. gonorrhoeae*

Dual infections with both *N. gonorrhoeae* and *C. trachomatis* are prevalent and it is generally recommended to do testing for both organisms. Specimens for *N. gonorrhoeae* should be collected prior to specimens for *C. trachomatis*.

■ **Pretest question #5:** The following statement is true. Collection of specimens for culture of *N. gonorrhoeae* should be obtained prior to specimens for culture of *C. trachomatis*.

METHOD A: IMMEDIATE, DIRECT PLATING OF SPECIMENS

Immediate plating of specimens is recommended to enhance recovery of the organism.

1. Insert the vaginal speculum, which has been moistened with warm **water**, into the patient's vagina. (Do not use any other lubricant because other substances may kill the organism.)

■ **Pretest question #2:** The following statement is false. The vaginal speculum used for visualizing the vagina and cervix should be moistened with a water-soluble gel so as to avoid any interference with specimen collection.

2. Using a large cotton swab, remove vaginal secretions and cervical exudate from the exocervix. Discard the cleaning swab.
3. Insert a sterile swab in the patient's cervical os until the tip is no longer visible (approximately 2 cm). A sterile cotton swab may be used if the plates are inoculated immediately after specimen collection. If a transport medium is used, calcium alginate or dacron swabs should be used for specimen collection.
4. Rotate the swab for 10 to 30 seconds.
5. Carefully remove the swab from the cervical os. Do not touch the vaginal walls while removing the swab.

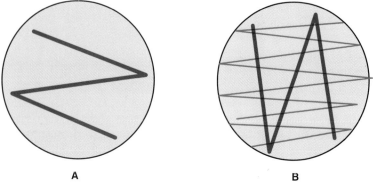

A   B

FIGURE 6-1

(**A**) and (**B**): Inoculation of Thayer-Martin media for the isolation of *N. gonorrhoeae.*

6. Immediately streak a modified Thayer-Martin agar plate with the swab. The plate should be streaked by rolling the swab onto the media using a "Z" pattern (Fig. 6-1A). The swab should be rolled on the plate to ensure that all areas of the swab come in to contact with the plate. Discard the swab.

7. Turn the plate 90 degrees and cross streak the entire plate with a second, clean sterile swab (Figure 6-1B). Discard the swab.

8. Place the inoculated media (agar side up) into a carbon dioxide-rich environment such as a CO_2 incubator or candle jar (Fig. 6-2).

    A candle jar is a glass container with a resealable lid. A candle is placed in the jar on top of the plates. The candle is lit and the jar is sealed. As the candle burns, oxygen is decreased and CO_2 increased (Fig. 6-3).

    Plates should be incubated at 35°C or held at room temperature. They should not be refrigerated or exposed to extreme temperatures.

■ **Pretest question #7:** Steps for handling an inoculated Thayer-Martin plate are as follows:

a. Place the inoculated plate (agar side up) into a carbon dioxide rich environment such as a CO_2 incubator or candle jar.

b. Maintain the temperature of the incubator at 35°C or hold the candle jar at room temperature.

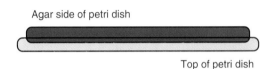

FIGURE 6-2
Incubation of culture plates.

METHOD B: USE OF TRANSPORT SYSTEMS

If immediate, direct plating is not possible, transport systems should be used to transport the specimen to the laboratory. Good results may be obtained using transport systems if the manufacturer's instructions are followed.

1. Follow steps 1 through 5 as described in Method A.
2. Immediately place swab in transport media. *N. gonorrhoeae* is very sensitive to drying. Swabs should not be allowed to dry out before processing.
3. Transport the specimens to the laboratory as soon as possible.
4. Specimens should not be refrigerated or exposed to extreme temperatures.

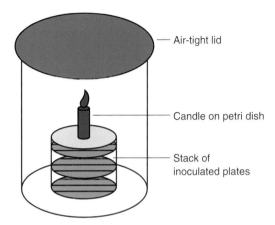

FIGURE 6-3
Candle jar.

The recovery of N. *gonorrhoeae* is increased if two sites, such as the endocervix and rectum, or two consecutive endocervical specimens are cultured. If obtaining an additional endocervical swab for culture of N. *gonorrhoeae*, insert the second swab 1 cm deeper into the cervical os than the previous swab.

Specimen Collection for Culture of *Chlamydia trachomatis*

Chlamydia trachomatis is an obligate intracellular organism found in columnar or cuboidal epithelial cells. Isolation of the organism is dependent upon removal of any endocervical exudate so as to obtain epithelial cells. When testing for both N. *gonorrhoeae* and C. *trachomatis*, two separate swabs (or one swab and one cytobrush) are needed. Cultures for N. *gonorrhoeae* should be done prior to cultures for C. *trachomatis*.

Tissue culture for C. *trachomatis* is difficult and not performed in many laboratories. A number of antigen detection methods are commercially available and used in place of tissue culture. Enzyme immunoassay (EIA), direct fluorescent antibody (DFA), and DNA probes are all used for the diagnosis of infection with *Chlamydia trachomatis*. Newer methods, such as polymerase chain reaction (PCR) and ligase chain reaction have a greater sensitivity than EIA, DFA, or DNA probes and are being used with increased frequency. Each of these commercially available tests contains specimen collection supplies and instructions. Be sure to be familiar with the testing procedure used in your laboratory. Use the collection and handling techniques appropriate for the test method that is in use.

The single most important aspect of specimen collection for C. *trachomatis* testing is to obtain an adequate number of cuboidal or columnar epithelial cells. Using a cytology brush rather than a swab may increase the number of epithelial cells collected, thus increasing the sensitivity of chlamydial testing.

1. Insert the vaginal speculum, which has been moistened with warm **water**, into the patient's vagina. (Do not use any other lubricant because other substances may kill the organism.)

2. Using a large cotton swab, remove vaginal secretions and cervical exudate from the exocervix. Discard the cleaning swab.
3. Insert a cytology brush or urogenital swab (calcium alginate or dacron swab on a wire or plastic shaft) in the patient's cervical os until the tip is no longer visible (approximately 2 cm). If specimens for *N. gonorrhoeae* have been collected, be sure to insert the swab or cytobrush 1 cm deeper than the previous swab.
4. Move the cytology brush from side to side, or if using a swab, rotate it for 10 to 30 seconds.
5. Carefully remove the brush or swab from the cervical os. Do not touch the vaginal walls while removing the swab.
6. Immediately place brush or swab in the transport media.
7. Transport the specimen to the laboratory as soon as possible. If there is a delay in transporting the specimen to the laboratory, it should be stored in the refrigerator.

Pretest question #8: Specimens for diagnosis of infection with *C. trachomatis* should be immediately placed into transport media and taken to the laboratory as soon as possible. If there is a delay in transport of the specimen, the transport media/specimen should be stored in the refrigerator.

URETHRAL SPECIMENS

Infection of the urethra (urethritis) may present with a variety of signs and symptoms including urethral or vaginal discharge, urinary frequency, dysuria, fever, and edema of the urinary meatus or vulva. Diagnosis of the specific cause of urethritis depends upon laboratory testing of appropriately collected specimens.

The most common types of urethritis are gonococcal urethritis caused by *N. gonorrhoeae* and nongonococcal urethritis, most frequently caused by *C. trachomatis*. Coexisting infections are prevalent and it is generally recommended to test for both *N. gonorrhoeae* and *C. trachomatis*.

Urethral infections are commonly diagnosed with a Gram stain and microbiological cultures. A Gram stain of a urethral discharge specimen can provide the clinician with valuable information regarding the cause of urethritis. Finding gram-negative intracellular (within polymorphonuclear cells) diplococci on a Gram stain of a urethral discharge is diagnostic for infection with *N. gonorrhoeae.* If polymorphonuclear cells are seen with no gram-negative diplococci, the most likely cause is *C. trachomatis.* A small number of smear-negative (no gram-negative diplococci seen on Gram stain) specimens, however, will be culture positive for *N. gonorrhoeae.* Therefore, if no gram-negative diplococci are seen, the specimen should be cultured for *N. gonorrhoeae.*

Less frequent causes of urethritis are *Candida albicans* and *Trichomonas vaginalis.* These organisms may be seen on a Gram stain of a urethral discharge but are best diagnosed using alternative methods. A saline wet mount can be examined for *T. vaginalis,* (see Chapter 4 for instructions on how to perform a saline wet mount); however, the wet mount is often negative in infected men. Diagnosis of *Trichomonas* infection in men is best accomplished by culturing the urethral discharge or first morning voided urine specimen. *C. albicans* may be diagnosed by either the saline wet mount or KOH preparation (see Chapter 4 for instructions on how to perform a saline wet mount or KOH preparation). A fungal culture for *C. albicans* may also be performed.

Specimen Collection

MALE SPECIMEN COLLECTION

1. Delay obtaining urethral specimens, ideally, until 1–2 hours after the patient has voided. Recent micturition may eliminate any urethral discharge, making visualization or isolation of the causative agent difficult.

■ **Pretest question #4:** The following statement is false. Urethral specimens for microbiological cultures should be obtained immediately after the individual has voided.

2. Have the patient "milk" the penis for several seconds. (While standing, the individual should place the thumb of one hand on the dorsal surface of the penis near the base. The index finger of the same hand should be placed on the ventral surface of the penis near the base. The person should then stroke the penis distally several times.)
3. Collect any visible exudate at the urethral meatus with 2 sterile swabs, one to be used for a Gram stain and one for

culture. A sterile cotton swab may be used if the plates and slides are inoculated immediately after specimen collection. If transport media are used, calcium alginate or Dacron swabs should be used for specimen collection.

4. If there is no obvious discharge, gently insert a urogenital swab (calcium alginate or dacron swab on a wire or plastic shaft) approximately 2 cm into the urethra. Rotate the swab in one direction for at least one revolution for 5 seconds.

5. Place the swab into the appropriate transport media or onto a Thayer-Martin agar plate. See steps 6–8 under endocervical specimens for the procedure on inoculation and incubation of Thayer-Martin plates. *N. gonorrhoeae* is very sensitive to drying. Swabs should not be allowed to dry out before processing.

6. A second swab should be collected for Gram staining. When collecting more than one swab, each successive swab should be inserted 1 cm deeper than the previous one. See p. 120 for instructions on Gram staining.

7. Repeat steps 4 and 5 to collect a specimen for laboratory testing for *C. trachomatis*.

8. Transport the specimens to the laboratory as soon as possible. Specimens for *N. gonorrhoeae* should not be refrigerated or exposed to extreme temperatures. Specimens for *C. trachomatis* should be stored in the refrigerator if there is a delay in transporting the specimen to the laboratory.

FEMALE SPECIMEN COLLECTION

In women, dysuria and urinary frequency are most often symptoms of cystitis. Patients presenting with these symptoms should be evaluated for cystitis. (See Chapter 3 for collection and handling of urine specimens for urinalysis and urine culture.) If urinalysis or urine culture results do not support the diagnosis of urinary tract infection, the patient may have urethritis rather than cystitis. In these cases a urethral specimen is examined for *N. gonorrhoeae* and *C. trachomatis*.

1. Delay obtaining urethral specimens, ideally, until 1–2 hours after the patient has voided. Recent micturition may eliminate any urethral discharge making visualization or isolation of the causative agent difficult.

2. With the patient in the lithotomy position, the clinician should gently "milk" (stroke) the anterior vaginal wall (proximally to distally) for a few seconds.
3. Gently insert a urogenital swab (calcium alginate or dacron swab on a wire or plastic shaft) approximately 2 cm into the urethra. Rotate the swab in one direction for at least one revolution for 5 seconds.
4. Place the swab into the appropriate transport media or onto a Thayer-Martin agar plate. See steps 6–8 under endocervical specimens for the procedure on inoculation and incubation of Thayer-Martin plates on page 154. *N. gonorrhoeae* is very sensitive to drying. Swabs should not be allowed to dry out before processing.
5. A second swab may be collected for Gram staining. See instructions on Gram staining on page 119. When collecting more than one swab, each successive swab should be inserted 1 cm deeper than the previous one.
6. Repeat steps 3 and 4 to collect a specimen for laboratory testing for *C. trachomatis*.
7. Transport the specimens to the laboratory as soon as possible. Specimens for *N. gonorrhoeae* should not be refrigerated or exposed to extreme temperatures. Specimens for *C. trachomatis* should be stored in the refrigerator if there is a delay in transporting the specimen to the laboratory.

▓▓▓▓ Clinical Tips

- Studies have shown that enhanced recovery of *N. gonorrhoeae* is facilitated if two sites, such as endocervix and rectum, or two consecutive endocervical specimens are cultured. (Baron et al., 1993; Mardh & Danielsson, 1990).
- Since some genital-tract pathogens are inhibited by cotton or components that may be present in wooden shafts, specimens should be collected on calcium alginate or dacron swabs on plastic or wire shafts.

▓ **Pretest question #3:** The following statement is true. Sterile Dacron swabs should be used for collecting endocervical specimens for microbiological culture of both *N. gonorrhoeae* and *C. trachomatis*.

- Thayer-Martin plates and transport media should be at room temperature when inoculated with the specimen.
- Always use fresh media. Check expiration dates on media and never use plates or tubes beyond the expiration date.
- *N. gonorrhoeae* are sensitive to drying, changes in temperature, or inadequate supply of CO_2. Therefore, inoculated plates should be immediately placed into a CO_2 environment and incubated at 35°C or held at room temperature. If placed in a candle jar, the jar should not be left at room temperature for longer than 1 to 2 hours. If transport media is used, swabs should be immediately placed in the transport media to avoid drying.
- Some strains of *N. gonorrhoeae* are inhibited by the antibiotics that are in Thayer-Martin media. The incidence of these susceptible strains vary by geographical and epidemiological factors. If sensitivity to the antibiotics in Thayer-Martin media is common, then both a selective (Thayer-Martin agar) and nonselective (chocolate agar) media should be inoculated.

CHAPTER 6 PRETEST ANSWERS

1. False. Direct smears (eg, Gram stains) of endocervical specimens lack specificity and sensitivity. Thus, the most accurate method for diagnosing cervicitis caused by *N. gonorrhoeae* is by culture.

2. False. Any lubricating agent other than **water** may interfere with laboratory testing. Thus, water is the only acceptable lubricating agent.

3. True. Some genital organisms are inhibited by cotton or components that may be present in wooden shafts. Specimens should be collected on sterile calcium alginate or Dacron swabs that are on plastic or wire shafts.

4. False. Urination can eliminate inflammatory discharges from the urethra and result in false negative culture results. Therefore, it is recommended that urethral specimens be taken 1 to 2 hours after the patient has voided.

5. True. Swabs for *N. gonorrhoeae* should be collected first as this organism is an extracellular pathogen present in the ex-

udate. *C. trachomatis* is an obligate intracellular organism found in columnar or cuboidal epithelial cells. It is therefore necessary to remove any exudate in order to obtain epithelial cells.

6. The answer is b. Discharge with more than 10 WBCs per HPF.

   a. The finding of 1–3 red blood cells may be a normal finding.

   c. Epithelial cells are a normal finding.

   d. A "fishy" or amine odor is consistent with a diagnosis of bacterial vaginosis. There is no cervical involvement with this infection.

7. After inoculation of a Thayer-Martin agar, one should:

   a. Place the inoculated plate (agar side up) into a carbon-dioxide rich environment such as a CO_2 incubator or candle jar.

   b. Maintain the temperature of the incubator at 35°C or hold the candle jar at room temperature.

8. If there is a delay in transport of the specimens for culture of *C. trachomatis*, the transport media/specimen should be stored in the refrigerator.

CHAPTER 6 POSTTEST

1. What are the two organisms that most commonly cause urethritis or cervicitis?

2. What three environmental factors are important to consider when handling specimens for isolation of *N. gonorrhoeae*?

3. What is the most important aspect of specimen collection for the diagnosis of chlamydial infections?

Questions 4–5: Multiple choice. Select the one best answer.

4. Regarding the collection and handling of endocervical specimens, which one of the following is **least** accurate?

   a. The culture or transport media used for isolation of bacteria that cause cervicitis/urethritis should be brought to room temperature before inoculation.

   b. If a Gram stain for GC is to be performed, two specimens should be collected. One swab should be used for Gram stain and one for culture.

   c. Recovery of *N. gonorrhoeae* is enhanced if a combined endocervical-vaginal specimen is obtained.

   d. A cytobrush should be used to obtain endocervical specimens for culture of *C. trachomatis*.

5. Newer laboratory tests (eg, Enzyme immunoassays and DNA probes) are replacing cultures for *N. gonorrhoeae* and *C. trachomatis* because:

   a. They are more sensitive and specific than microbiological cultures.

   b. They are faster and more convenient than microbiological cultures.

   c. They require a less-invasive diagnostic approach than do microbiological cultures.

   d. Specimen collection is easier and may be done in the individual's home as well as in a clinical practice setting.

Questions 6–8: In the diagnosis of infectious diseases, it is important to be aware of the laboratory testing procedures that are available and appropriate for diagnostic purposes. From the lettered list below, choose the most appropriate laboratory test for effective diagnosis of the numbered conditions.

   a. Microbiological culture

   b. Gram stain

   c. Enzyme immunoassay

   d. Saline wet mount

   e. Polymerase chain reaction (PCR)

6. Cervicitis caused by *N. gonorrhoeae*

7. Vaginitis caused by *T. vaginalis*

8. Urethritis caused by *N. gonorrhoeae*

CHAPTER 6 POSTTEST ANSWERS

1. The two organisms most commonly causing urethritis or cervicitis are *N. gonorrhoeae* and *C. trachomatis*

2. *N. gonorrhoeae* is very sensitive to drying, temperature, and CO_2 concentration.

3. *C. trachomatis* is an obligate intracellular parasite found in cuboidal or columnar epithelial cells. Therefore, the most important aspect of specimen collection is to obtain an adequate number of epithelial cells. This requires removing any exudate and using a cytobrush to gently scrape the mucosal surface of the endocervix.

4. The answer is c. *N. gonorrhoeae* does not thrive in the vagina (except in prepubescent girls). Thus, obtaining a vaginal specimen will not enhance recovery of the organism.

5 The answer is b. The newer technologies are generally faster and more convenient than microbiological culture.

6. The answer is a, microbiological culture. Gram stains of endocervical specimens lack sensitivity and specificity. Therefore, a culture must be done to diagnose cervicitis caused by *N. gonorrhoeae*.

7. The answer is d, saline wet mount. Vaginitis caused by *T. vaginalis* may be diagnosed by the saline wet mount. It is important that the specimen be examined within 15 minutes of collection to ensure the motility of the organism that is needed for identification.

8. The answer is b. Gram stain. The Gram stain is a fast, accurate, cost-effective method used in the diagnosis of urethritis caused by *N. gonorrhoeae*. If the Gram stain does not show gram-negative diplococci, then a culture should be done to rule out gonorrhea definitively.

REFERENCES

Baron, E. J., Cassell, G. H., Duffy, L. B., Eschenbach, D. A., Greenwood, J. R., Harvey, S. M., Madinger, N. E., Peterson, E. M., & Waites, K. B. (1993). Laboratory diagnosis of female genital tract infections. *Cumitech 17A*. Washington, DC: American Society for Microbiology.

Mardh, P. A. & Danielsson, D. (1990). *Neisseria gonorrhoeae*. In K. K. Holmes et al. (Eds.), *Sexually transmitted diseases* (2nd ed.), pp. 903–916. New York: McGraw Hill.

SUGGESTED READINGS

Centers for Disease Control and Prevention (CDC) (1993). Recommendations for the prevention and management of *Chlamydia trachomatis* infections, 1993. *Morbidity and Mortality Weekly Report, 42*(RR-12), 1–39.

McCormack, W. M., & Rein, M. F. (1995). Urethritis. In G. L. Mandell, J. E. Bennett, & F. Dolin (Eds.). *Principles and practice of infectious diseases* (4th ed.). (pp. 1063–1074). New York: Churchill Livingstone.

Pasteorek II, J. G. (1994). *Obstetric and gynecologic infectious disease*. New York: Raven Press.

Rein, M. F. (1995). Vulvovaginits and cervicitis. In G.L. Mandell, J. E. Bennett, & F. Dolin (Eds.). *Principles and practice of infectious diseases* (4th ed.), pp. 1075–1090. New York: Churchill Livingstone.

Sweet, R. L., & Gibbs, R. S., (1995). *Infectious diseases of the female genital tract* (3rd ed.). Baltimore: Williams and Wilkins.

Wallach, J. (1996). *Interpretation of diagnostic tests: A synopsis of laboratory medicine* (6th ed.). Boston: Little, Brown and Company.

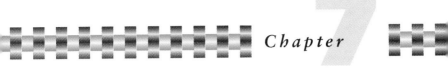

Miscellaneous Microscopic Examinations

Primary care clinicians perform many different microscopic examinations on specimens obtained from their patients. The Clinical Laboratory Improvement Amendment of 1988 (CLIA'88) regulates the type of microscopic examinations that may be done by advanced practice nurses, physicians, and other health care practitioners (see Chapter 1). These microscopic examinations are called provider performed microscopy (PPM) tests and include examination of urine sediment (Chapter 3), saline wet mount and potassium-hydroxide (KOH) preparations of vaginal secretions (Chapter 4), fecal leukocyte determinations, KOH on skin or nail scrapings for the diagnosis of fungal infections, ferning test for the evaluation of premature rupture of fetal membranes (PROM), and examination for pinworm ova.

This chapter will provide the reader with instructions on how to perform and interpret a fecal leukocyte examination, KOH mount on skin and nail scrapings, ferning test, and examination for pinworm ova.

OBJECTIVES

Upon completion of this chapter, the reader will be able to:

1. Describe the proper technique for the collection and handling of specimens for fecal leukocyte determination.

OBJECTIVES (Continued)

2. Perform and interpret a microscopic examination for fecal leukocytes.
3. Describe the proper technique for the collection and handling of skin and nail scrapings for the identification of fungal elements.
4. Perform and interpret a KOH mount on skin or nail scrapings.
5. Describe the proper technique for the collection and handling of vaginal specimens for the identification of patients with PROM.
6. Perform and interpret a microscopic examination of fluids for the identification of patients with PROM.
7. Describe the proper technique for the collection and handling of specimens for the detection and identification of pinworm ova.
8. Perform and interpret a microscopic examination for the detection and identification of pinworm ova.

Please take the pretest. After completing the pretest, read the material in the chapter.

CHAPTER 7 PRETEST

Questions 1–4: Answer true or false.

1. The ideal portion of the fecal specimen to inspect for leukocytes is the central-most area of the fecal material.

2. Collection of specimens for the diagnosis of premature rupture of fetal membranes should include both vaginal and cervical secretions.

3. Skin infections with dermatophytes are diagnosed by seeing hyphae in a KOH mount of scrapings from lesions.

4. If no leukocytes are present on microscopic examination of a fecal specimen, the clinician should then send the specimen for culture for bacterial enteric pathogens.

Questions 5–7: Fill in the blank.

5. The normal pH of amniotic fluid is between _____.

6. The two medically important types of fungi are _____ and _____.

7. At what time of day should specimens for detection of pinworm ova be collected?

The pretest answers will appear throughout the text of the chapter and before the posttest.

MICROSCOPIC EXAMINATION FOR FECAL LEUKOCYTES

Acute diarrhea is a common complaint of patients seen in a primary care office. Infectious diarrheal disease can be classified as either inflammatory or noninflammatory. The noninflammatory diarrheas are most commonly caused by viruses. They are self-limited, and can be treated with simple oral rehydration therapy. Inflammatory diarrheas are generally more serious and require culture for bacterial enteric pathogens and may require antibiotic treatment.

Stool examination for white blood cells (WBCs; leukocytes) is a rapid test that can easily be performed in the office laboratory and can be helpful in the differentiation of noninflammatory from inflammatory syndromes. Inflammatory enterocolitis causes damage to the mucosal lining, which results in the presence of WBCs in the fecal specimen. Most of the WBCs present will be polymorphonuclear cells (polys, PMNs, or neutrophils).

In the diagnosis of enterocolitis, a fecal leukocyte determination should be done if:

- Diarrhea is severe, bloody, or lasts longer than 2–3 days.
- Patients have recently traveled to an area where parasites or bacterial pathogens are endemic.
- Patients have a history of eating unpasteurized or poorly refrigerated dairy products.
- Patients have a history of eating improperly cooked or poorly handled poultry products.

If WBCs are seen in the fecal specimen, a stool culture should be ordered for enteric pathogens. Based on the culture results, antibiotic therapy should be considered. If no WBCs are seen, the etiology is most likely viral and cultures may not be necessary.

At best, the sensitivity of fecal leukocyte determinations is 60% to 70%. Therefore, in patients with signs and symptoms of an inflammatory enterocolitis, in whom the presence of an enteric bacterial pathogen must be ruled out with some degree of certainty, (immunocompromised, elderly, etc.) bacterial cultures should be done regardless of the fecal leukocyte result.

Specimen Collection

Patients should collect a fresh stool sample in a clean specimen container. If necessary, the clinician can palpate the rectum and collect fecal material from the glove into a clean specimen container. A rectal swab is not an adequate specimen for fecal leukocyte determination, as results from rectal swabs are often falsely negative.

Fecal leukocyte tests should be done on fresh specimens because many components in the fecal specimen can disintegrate WBCs. Therefore, examination of the specimen should be done as soon as possible. If the specimen cannot be examined right away, it should be stored at room temperature until the test can be done.

Specimen Processing

MATERIALS

- Microscope slide and coverslip
- Cotton swab
- Methylene blue stain
- Brightfield microscope

PROCEDURE

1. Examine the specimen for mucus or areas containing gross blood. The areas of the specimen containing mucus or red blood cells (RBCs) are more likely to have WBCs. These areas are usually located on the outside of the stool specimen. Using a cotton swab, remove a small amount of stool containing mucus or RBCs.

■ **Pretest question #1:** The following statement is false. The ideal area of the fecal specimen to inspect for leukocytes is the central-most area of the fecal material.

2. Place a small sample on a clean microscope slide.
3. Add 1 to 2 drops of methylene blue stain to the sample and mix thoroughly.
4. Place a coverslip over the specimen/methylene blue mixture and allow the slide to sit for 2 minutes.
5. Examine the slide using 40× objective for the presence of WBCs. Fecal specimens contain a significant amount of debris (food particles, bacteria, etc.) and therefore, leukocytes may be difficult to see. Estimate the number of WBCs present per high-power field (Fig. 7-1).

Interpretation

The presence of WBCs in a fecal specimen indicates inflammation of the intestinal mucosa. This may be caused by invasive pathogens such as *Salmonella, Shigella,* or *Campylobacter* or inflammatory conditions such as ulcerative colitis or antibiotic-associated

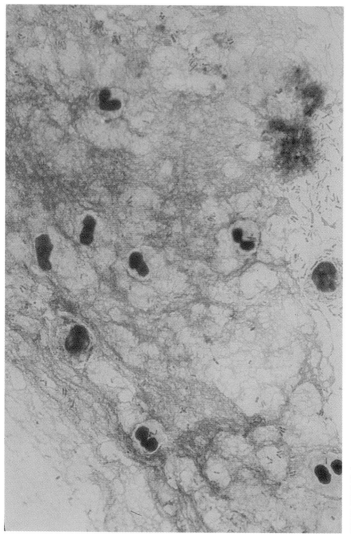

FIGURE 7-1
Positive fecal leukocytes (400×).

colitis. If WBCs are present, the stool specimen should be sent for culture for enteric pathogens.

A problem with the fecal leukocyte determination is that it has not been standardized and various methods are used. Also, there is no one defined positive test result. Some procedures use positive cut-off values of 5 or 10 leukocytes per high-power field and others consider any leukocytes present as a positive result. Several studies have shown that the fecal leukocyte determination is lacking in both specificity and sensitivity and results should always be correlated with the clinical picture when assessing the need for culture.

If no fecal leukocytes are seen, it generally indicates a noninvasive diarrhea, most likely of viral etiology, and a culture may not be necessary.

Pretest question #4: The following statement is false. If no leukocytes are present on microscopic examination of a fecal specimen, the clinician should then send the specimen for culture for bacterial enteric pathogens.

Alternatives to Microscopy for the Determination of Fecal Leukocytes

The microscopic test for determining fecal leukocytes has never been standardized and can be very difficult to interpret because of the large amount of debris in stool specimens. Recently, latex agglutination tests for determining the presence of WBCs in fecal specimens have become available. These tests are easier to interpret and specimens may be stored for prolonged periods of time before testing. As with all commercially available testing protocols, adhere to the manufacturers instructions and never use expired reagents.

POTASSIUM HYDROXIDE (KOH) MOUNT ON SKIN OR NAIL SCRAPINGS

Fungi may cause infections on skin, nails, hair, or mucosal surfaces, such as the vaginal tract or mouth. The diagnosis of fungal infections can often be accomplished by visualizing fungal elements on scrapings from infected lesions. A solution of 10%

potassium hydroxide is added to the specimen to dissolve cells and debris, thus making the fungal elements more easily seen. See Chapter 4 for instructions on performing KOH mounts on vaginal specimens.

Specimen Collection and Processing

MATERIALS

- Microscope slide and coverslip
- Scraping instrument:
  ∘ Sterile scalpel blade
  ∘ Edge of microscope slide that has been surface disinfected with 70% alcohol.
  ∘ Tongue blade, etc.
- Alcohol lamp or other heat source.
- 10% KOH reagent: Available from laboratory supply companies or may be prepared by dissolving 10 grams of KOH crystals in 80 mL of distilled water and 10 mL of glycerin. Nail scrapings or thick skin scrapings may require a stronger alkaline (20% KOH) reagent. The clearing capabilities of the KOH may also be enhanced by using 40% aqueous dimethyl sulfoxide (DMSO) reagent in place of distilled water to dissolve the KOH crystals.
- A small amount of dye may be added to the KOH reagent to enhance visualization of fungal elements. The dyes that are commonly used are lactophenol cotton blue and chlorazol E Black.
- Sterile gauze. Cotton swabs should not be used for cleansing as they may leave fibers that can be confused with hyphae.
- 70% alcohol
- Brightfield microscope

PROCEDURES

Skin Scrapings

1. Clean skin lesions with soap and water to remove dirt, oil, and any cosmetics or lotions. After washing with soap and water, cleanse the area with gauze that has been soaked in 70% alcohol. Be sure to remove any remaining soap.

2. Scrape the peripheral area of a lesion with a sterile knife blade or edge of an alcohol disinfected microscope slide. Scrapings should be fairly deep and from the active, outer border of the lesions. The central area of the lesion generally will not contain fungal elements (Fig. 7-2). Scaly lesions should be scraped and the top of vesicles or pustules should be cut for examination.
3. Place the scrapings in the center of a clean glass microscope slide.
4. Add a drop of KOH reagent and cover with a coverslip. Gently press the coverslip down on the sample.
5. Heat gently (**DO NOT BOIL**) by passing the slide through a flame four or five times.
6. Examine the slide with the low-power (10×) objective for the presence of hyphae, spores, or yeast. Confirm possible fungal elements with the high-power (40×) objective. This is a wet-mount preparation and, therefore, the condenser should be raised and the aperture diaphragm should be closed. See Chapter 2 for detailed instructions on how to use the microscope.

Thicker specimens may require additional time for the KOH to dissolve the epithelial cells. The slide may sit at room temperature for 5–15 minutes to allow clearing of thicker specimens.

Nail Scrapings

1. Scales on the surface of the nail, or between the nail and the nail bed should be collected by scraping with a knife blade. The most desirable material for examination is the waxy, subungual debris. It may be necessary to remove a portion of the nail with nail clippers in order to sample the infected area. Nail clippings are not ideal for KOH preps or fungal culture. If clippings are used, they should be ground or minced before processing.
2. Follow steps 3–6 of the procedure for skin scrapings. Nail scrapings may take longer to clear than skin scrapings.

Oral Lesions

1. The white membranous lesions of oral *Candida* infection (thrush) are scraped with a tongue blade. These lesions are

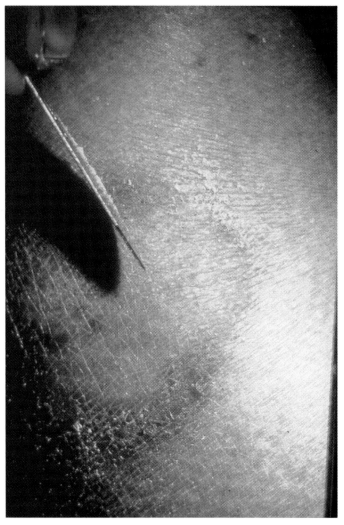

FIGURE 7-2
Ringworm lesion.

generally adherent and painful. When scraped, they may bleed and reveal an inflamed, erythematous base.

2. Follow steps 3–6 of the procedure for skin scrapings.

Interpretation

The KOH preparation is examined with the low-power and high-power objectives for fungal elements.

The fungi of medical importance have two forms:

- Molds, which grow in long, branching, threadlike filaments called hyphae and reproduce by producing spores (Fig. 7-3). Hyphae generally have parallel sides and may have cross-walls called septae (Fig. 7-3C).
- Yeast, which are single-celled organisms and reproduce by budding. **Note:** *Candida albicans* can elongate to form structures called pseudohyphae. Pseudohyphae are formed only by *C. albicans* and indicate tissue invasion (see Fig. 7-3).

Pretest question #6. The two medically important types of fungi are yeast and molds.

The fungi that infect the skin, hair, and nails are called dermatophytes and infections with these agents are called dermatophytoses. Common terms to describe these infections are ringworm (tinea corporis), athlete's foot (tinea pedis), and jock itch (tinea cruris). KOH mounts show hyphae and may or may not show spores (Fig. 7-4).

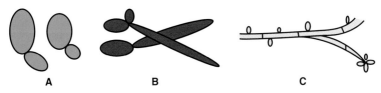

A　　　　**B**　　　　**C**

FIGURE 7-3
(**A**) Budding yeast cells. (**B**) Pseudohyphae. (**C**) Septate hyphae and spores.

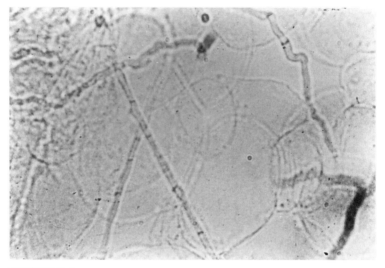

FIGURE 7-4
Positive KOH mount showing hyphae (400×).

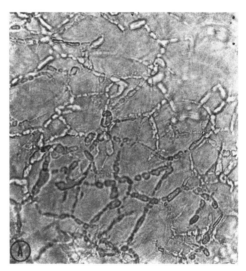

FIGURE 7-5
"Mosaic" pattern in KOH preparation (400×).

■ **Pretest question #3.** The following statement is true. Skin infections with dermatophytes are diagnosed by seeing true hyphae in a KOH mount of scrapings from lesions.

Tinea versicolor (pityriasis versicolor) is a superficial infection of the skin caused by the fungus *Malassezia furfur.* The KOH mounts of skin scrapings will show many small spores and hyphal fragments ("spaghetti and meatballs") (Fig. 7-6).

Scrapings of oral lesions for the diagnosis of Candidiasis (thrush) will show budding yeast cells with pseudohyphae (see Fig. 4-3). Scrapings of oral lesions may also be Gram stained (see Chapter 5 and Fig. 5-7).

Clinical Tips

- In skin scrapings, epidermal cells may not fully dissolve and the edges of the cells may look like hyphae.
- Cholesterol crystals and other debris may deposit around epidermal cells in a "mosaic" pattern. This mosaic is often misidentified as fungal hyphae (Fig. 7-5). The mosaic may be differentiated from hyphae by its abrupt changes in width

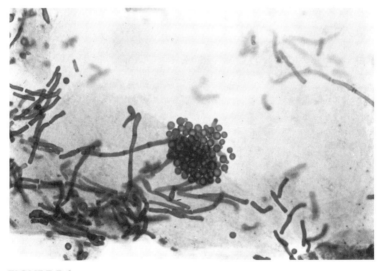

FIGURE 7-6
Positive KOH mount, tinea versicolor. A stain has been added to the KOH to enhance visualization of the fungal elements (400×).

and the way in which it appears to surround some cells completely.

- Lint or cotton fibers may be confused with hyphae. These contaminants generally have thick edges and do not have crosswalls.
- Finding a few budding yeast cells in a KOH preparation must be interpreted with caution. Small numbers of yeast, including *C. albicans,* may be found as normal skin, vaginal, or oral flora. More reliable than the finding of budding yeast cells is the finding of pseudohyphae. The pseudohyphal form of *C. albicans* is associated with adherence to and invasion of tissue.

THE FERN TEST FOR THE DETERMINATION OF PREMATURE RUPTURE OF FETAL MEMBRANES (PROM)

The fern test is a fast and simple test that can be used in pregnant women to aid in the diagnosis of PROM. PROM is defined as rupture of the fetal membranes before the onset of labor. The identification of PROM is important because of the fetal and maternal complications associated with this condition. The main complications are premature labor and delivery, maternal and/or fetal infections, and umbilical cord compression or prolapse.

Specimen Collection and Processing

MATERIALS

- Sterile cotton swab
- Microscope slide
- pH paper (range 4.5 to 7.5)
- Brightfield microscope

PROCEDURE

1. Insert vaginal speculum, which has been moistened with warm **water**, into the patient's vagina. Do not use any other lubricant, because other lubricants may interfere with slide analysis.

2. Collect a sample of fluid from the vaginal fornix onto a sterile cotton swab. Care must be taken to avoid the cervix, because cervical mucus will give a false-positive result.

Pretest question #2: The following statement is false. Collection of specimens for the diagnosis of premature rupture of fetal membranes should include both vaginal and cervical secretions.

3. Touch the specimen swab on a strip of pH paper, then roll the swab on a clean glass microscope slide, creating a thin film. Set the slide aside to air dry.
4. Immediately examine the pH paper and compare the color to the color chart provided.
5. Allow the slide to dry completely before examining it under the microscope. Air drying the slide for a minimum of 10 minutes is the preferred method of slide preparation. This method has been shown to increase the sensitivity of the test over flame drying or drying for only 3 minutes (Bennett, 1993).
6. Examine the slide under low power without a coverslip for the typical arborization or ferning pattern.

Interpretation

Positive: Amniotic fluid has a pH between 7.0 and 7.5. A typical crystallization pattern is observed on microscopic examination (Fig. 7-7).

Negative: Normal vaginal pH during pregnancy: 4.5 to 6.0. There is no evidence of ferning.

Pretest question #5: The normal pH of amniotic fluid is between 7.0 and 7.5.

Clinical Tips

- Alkaline pH and ferning are not specific for amniotic fluid. Other fluids, such as blood, cervical mucus, semen, and some urine specimens, can cause crystallization to occur or a pH greater than 7.0 (false positive).

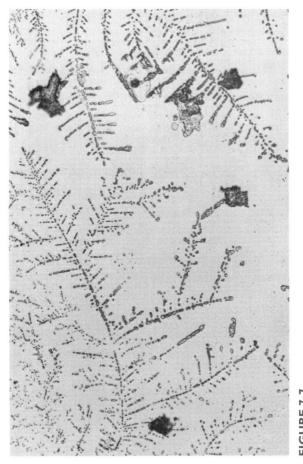

FIGURE 7-7
Positive fern test.

■ Prolonged rupture of membranes (> 24 hours) or slow, minimal leaks can give false negative results both in the pH determination and fern test.

EXAMINATION FOR PINWORM OVA

Enterobius vermicularis (pinworm) is found worldwide and is one of the most common parasitic infections in children. At night, the adult female worm migrates from the anus to the perianal area where she lays her eggs. Because the eggs are deposited outside the intestinal tract, examination of stool specimens for pinworm ova is often negative. The procedure most commonly used for the diagnosis of pinworm infection is the cellophane tape method.

Specimen Collection

MATERIALS

Provide the patient or parent of the patient with enough material to collect from three to five consecutive morning specimens.

- Collection kits (paddles or strips) for pinworm examination are commercially available and widely used.
- Microscope slide
- Gloves

Clinical Tip

■ If a commercially available product is not used, a collection device can be made by placing a looped strip of cellophane tape (adhesive side out) on one end of a tongue depressor. **Do not use frosted tape, use regular, clear cellophane tape.** This gives a sticky layer of tape that can be pressed to the perianal skin for specimen collection. See Figure 7–8A. The procedure below is written for use with the homemade collection device. If using a commercially prepared product, follow the instructions and recommendations of the manufacturer.

PROCEDURE

Specimens should be obtained in the morning before the patient has bathed or gone to the bathroom. Patients, or the parents of

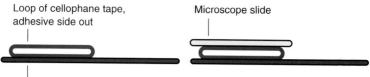

Loop of cellophane tape,
adhesive side out

Microscope slide

Tongue blade

FIGURE 7-8
(**A**) Pinworm paddle before collection. (**B**) Pinworm paddle after collection.

patients (if children), should be given collection materials and instructions on the proper methods of specimen collection.

■ **Pretest question #7:** Specimens for detection of pinworm ova should be collected in the morning.

Three to five consecutive morning specimens should be examined. All collection material may be given to the patient or parent and returned to the laboratory after the final sample is collected.

Pinworms are transmitted by the fecal-oral route. Advise the person collecting the specimen to wear gloves and to wash his or her hands well. The person performing the microscopic examination should also wear gloves to prevent transmission of the organism.

1. With one hand separate the buttocks to expose the anus.
2. Hold the collection device in the other hand with the sticky side out. Firmly press the adhesive surface against the perianal areas. Sample the skin of the entire circular area around the anus.
3. After collection of the specimen, press the microscope slide on top of the sticky surface (see Fig. 7-8B).
4. Place the entire collection device into a bag or envelope and return it to the office or laboratory.
5. Wash hands thoroughly after specimen collection.

Specimen Processing

MATERIALS

- Brightfield microscope
- Xylene
- Gloves

PROCEDURE

1. Using scissors, remove the tongue blade from the microscope slide by cutting the cellophane tape that is attached to the tongue blade. The tape attached to the microscope slide should remain (Fig. 7-9).

2. Using forceps, lift one edge of the tape that is attached to the microscope slide and place 1 small drop of xylene on the slide under the raised tape. Gently press the tape down onto the microscope slide. The xylene will clear the adhesive, enhancing detection and identification of pinworm ova.

Clinical Tip

■ Xylene fumes can be toxic. Avoid prolonged exposure to fumes and use in a well-ventilated area.

3. Examine the specimen with the low-power objective (10×). This is a wet-mount preparation; therefore, the condenser should be raised and the aperture diaphragm should be closed. (See Chapter 2 for detailed instructions on how to use the microscope.) If pinworm ova are seen with the low-power objective, confirm their identity using the high-power (40×) objective.

Interpretation

Pinworm ova are large (50–60 µm long—about the same size as a squamous epithelial cell), and football shaped, with one slightly flattened side. The developing larva may be seen inside the egg shell (Fig. 7-10).

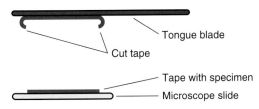

FIGURE 7-9
Preparation of a slide for microscopic examination.

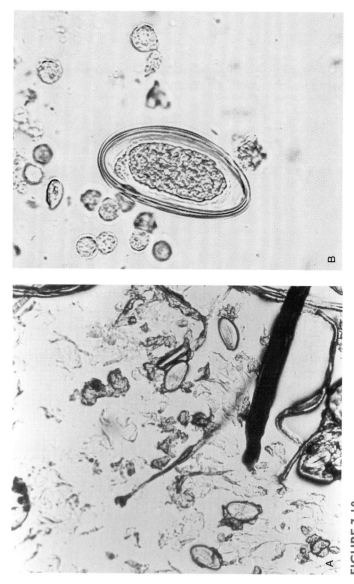

FIGURE 7-10
Pinworm ova (**A**) 100× (**B**) 400×.

▓▓▓ Clinical Tips

- It is unusual to see the adult worm when doing the cellophane tape test. Lint or threads may be present on the slide and should not be mistaken for worms.
- A single negative test result does not rule out infection. A series of three to five negative tests should be obtained to exclude a diagnosis of pinworm infection.

CHAPTER 7 PRETEST ANSWERS

1. False. Fecal leukocytes are generally found in mucus on the outside of the fecal specimen.

2. False. Cervical mucus may cause a false-positive ferning test.

3. True

4. False. If fecal leukocytes are not seen on microscopic examination, it most likely indicates a viral diarrhea; and therefore, culture for bacterial pathogens may not be indicated.

5. The normal pH of amniotic fluid is between 7.0 and 7.5.

6. The two medically important types of fungi are yeast and molds.

7. Specimens for detection of pinworm ova should be collected in the morning, before the individual has bathed or gone to the bathroom.

CHAPTER 7 POSTTEST

1. Which stain is used in the fecal leukocyte test?

2. What is the significance of seeing many WBCs in a fecal specimen?

3. Describe the procedure for collecting skin scrapings for a KOH preparation.

4. Name three substances or fluids that can cause a false-positive ferning test.

5. Describe the identifying characteristics of pinworm ova.

Questions 6–9: Answer true or false.

6. A rectal swab specimen may be used for detecting the presence of fecal leukocytes.

7. In the fern test, gentle heating of the slide will increase the sensitivity of the test.

8. Seeing yeast with pseudohyphae on a KOH preparation of scrapings from oral lesions indicates infection with *C. albicans*.

9. *Enterobius vermicularis* is a sexually transmitted parasite that most commonly affects young, sexually active adults.

CHAPTER 7 POSTTEST ANSWERS

1. Methylene blue is the stain used in the fecal leukocyte test.

2. Many WBCs in a stool specimen indicates mucosal invasion. This could be caused by an invasive pathogen such as *Salmonella, Shigella,* or *Campylobacter* or inflammatory conditions such as ulcerative colitis or antibiotic-associated colitis.

3. Skin lesions should be cleaned with soap and water, then wiped with alcohol. The outer border of the cleaned lesions should be scraped with a blade or edge of a microscope slide.

4. The substances that can cause a false positive ferning test are cervical mucus, blood, semen, and urine.

5. The distinguishing characteristics of pinworm ova are: large size (30–50 µm in length), football shaped, and one flattened end.

6. False. Rectal swab specimens often result in falsely negative results. Patients should collect fresh specimens in a clean container or, alternatively, from the clinician's glove after a rectal examination.

7. False. When performing the fern test, the slide should be allowed to air dry for at least 10 minutes.

8. True. Budding yeast with pseudohyphae are characteristic of *C. albicans.*

9. False. *E. vermicularis* is transmitted by the fecal-oral route and is most commonly found in young children.

REFERENCES

Bennett, S. L., Cullen, J. B., Sherrer, D. M., & Woods, J. R. (1993). The ferning and nitrazine tests of amniotic fluid between 12 and 41 weeks gestation. *American Journal of Perinatology, 10*, 101–104.

SUGGESTED READINGS

Baron, E. J., Peterson, L. R., & Finegold, S. M. (Eds.). (1994). *Diagnostic microbiology* (9th ed.). St. Louis: Mosby.

Garite, T. J., & Spellacy, W. N. (1994). Premature rupture of membranes. In J. R. Scott et al. (Eds.), *Danforth's obstetrics and gynecology* (7th ed.), pp. 305–308. Philadelphia: J. B. Lippincott.

Haan, H. H., Offermans, J. P., Smits, F., Schouten, H. J., & Peeters, L. L. (1994). Value of the fern test to confirm or reject the diagnosis of ruptured membranes is modest in nonlaboring women presenting with nonspecific vaginal fluid loss. *American Journal of Perinatology, 11*, 46–50.

Murray, P. R., Baron, E. J., Pfaller, M. A., Tenover, F. C., & Yolken, R. H. (Eds.) (1995). *Manual of clinical microbiology* (6th ed.). Washington, DC: American Society for Microbiology.

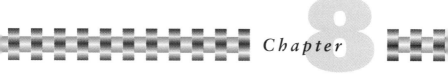

Diagnosis of Streptococcal Pharyngitis

Pharyngitis is one of the most common conditions seen by primary care providers. There are many infectious causes of pharyngitis, the most common being viruses (eg, adenoviruses, Epstein-Barr virus). A very important bacterial cause of pharyngitis is *Streptococcus pyogenes* (Group A streptococci). Group A streptococci account for 5%–30% of all cases of pharyngitis. Streptococcal pharyngitis is most prevalent in the pediatric population (5 to 15 years) and is associated with significant morbidity and occasionally serious sequelae such as rheumatic fever and acute glomerulonephritis.

In order to ensure proper treatment, clinicians must identify individuals with streptococcal pharyngitis. Proper antibiotic treatment will alleviate symptoms, prevent the spread of the disease, and is essential to prevent the development of rheumatic fever.

It is equally important to identify the individuals (70%–80%) with signs and symptoms of pharyngitis who do not have streptococcal pharyngitis and, therefore, do not require antibiotic treatment. There is always a risk associated with the administration of antibiotics. Side effects, allergies, and the alteration of the indigenous microflora are possible deleterious effects of antibiotic treatment. Inappropriate use of antibiotics has also led to an increase in the emergence of antibiotic-resistant organisms. Resistance to penicillin has developed in many oro- and nasopharyngeal organisms. This resistance may be due to the indiscriminate use of this antibiotic. At this time, there are no known strains of *S. pyogenes* resistant to penicillin, making penicillin the antibiotic of choice for treatment of streptococcal pharyngitis in those patients who are not allergic to penicillin.

The diagnosis of streptococcal pharyngitis is based on clinical and laboratory findings. Some clinical clues that an individual may have streptococcal pharyngitis are as follows:

- A red and edematous pharynx or tonsils
- A white to yellowish exudate on the tonsils or tonsilar crypts
- Cervical lymph nodes that are swollen and tender
- Fever
- No signs or symptoms of viral upper respiratory tract infection such as rhinitis, conjunctivitis, cough, or hoarseness

These signs and symptoms are relatively nonspecific, and clinical diagnosis of this infection is difficult even for experienced clinicians. Both the American Heart Association and American Academy of Pediatrics recommend laboratory testing of throat specimens for the definitive diagnosis of streptococcal pharyngitis. (For more detailed guidelines for determining the need for diagnostic testing for streptoccal pharyngitis, see Appendix: Case Studies Key, #5 [A, B, and C].)

OBJECTIVES

Upon completion of this chapter, the reader will be able to:

1. Describe the proper technique for the collection and handling of throat specimens for culture and rapid testing for Group A streptococci.
2. Perform and interpret a throat culture for Group A streptococci.
3. Recognize alpha and beta hemolysis on a sheep-blood agar plate.
4. Discuss methods for the identification of Group A streptococci.
5. Describe the advantages and disadvantages of the rapid antigen detection tests for Group A streptococci.
6. Correlate laboratory and clinical findings to diagnose the causes of pharyngitis.

Please take the pretest. After completing the pretest, read the material in the chapter.

CHAPTER 8 PRETEST

Questions 1–3: Answer true or false.

1. Group A streptococci produce beta hemolysis on a sheep-blood agar plate.

2. When streaking an agar plate with a throat swab for the diagnosis of streptococcal pharyngitis, the specimen swab should be rolled over the entire surface of the agar plate.

3. The throat culture is the "gold standard" for the diagnosis of streptococcal pharyngitis.

4. Describe the procedure for obtaining a throat swab from an individual presenting with signs and symptoms of pharyngitis.

Question 5: Multiple choice. Select the one best answer.

5. The preferred agar for the isolation and identification of Group A streptococci is:

   a. Sheep-blood agar

   b. Human-blood agar

   c. Horse-blood agar

   d. Agar plates without blood cells

The pretest answers will appear throughout the text of the chapter and before the posttest.

SPECIMEN COLLECTION

Depress the tongue completely with a tongue blade. Using a sterile Dacron swab, vigorously swab both tonsillar areas and the posterior pharyngeal wall. Be sure to swab any visible exudate. The posterior pharyngeal wall should be swabbed last, as this area is highly ennervated and swabbing may cause the patient to gag.

Pretest question #4: Describe the procedure for obtaining a throat swab from an individual presenting with signs and symptoms of pharyngitis.

After collection, the swab may be directly plated onto appropriate media or placed in a commercially available specimen collection tube that contains transport media. Always follow the manufacturer's instructions when using commercially prepared collection materials.

SPECIMEN PROCESSING

MATERIALS

- 5% Sheep-blood agar plate—sheep-blood agar plates are the preferred media for the isolation and identification of Group A streptococci.

Pretest question #5. The answer is a. The preferred agar for the isolation and identification of Group A streptococci is sheep-blood agar.

- Bacitracin differentiation disks (0.04 units per disk). This disk will inhibit the growth of group A beta-hemolytic streptococci, while other beta-hemolytic organisms will not be inhibited.
- Bacteriological loop
- Alcohol lamp or Bunsen burner
- Incubator (35°C)

PROCEDURE

1. Roll the swab over **one third** of a blood agar plate that has come to room temperature. The swab should be rotated

during inoculation to ensure that all sampled material is plated.

■ **Pretest question #2.** The following statement is false. When streaking an agar plate with a throat swab for the diagnosis of streptococcal pharyngitis, the specimen swab should be rolled over the entire surface of the agar plate.

2. With a sterile loop, streak out the specimen using the three quadrant technique (see pp. 202–203).
3. Incubate the plates aerobically at 35–37°C for 18–24 hours. After incubation, inspect the plates as described below.

Interpretation

After incubation, examine the plate for small (approximately 1 mm or less), transparent colonies surrounded by a zone of complete clearing of the red blood cells (RBCs); this is known as beta hemolysis.

Reading a throat culture plate can be difficult and requires experience and proper training. The normal flora of the throat includes many organisms, and these normal organisms must be differentiated from the Group A streptococci. In order to identify Group A streptococci properly you must be familiar with colony morphology and hemolytic reactions.

Colony Morphology

Bacterial colonies are usually described by the following categories:

- Size: Usually in millimeters
- Color: Gray, yellow, red, black, green, and so on
- Edge of colony: Circular, irregular, and so on
- Height and contour: Flat, raised, convex, and so on

Group A streptococci are small (<1 mm), transparent colonies. They may have a slightly gray color; however, most of the time, they are colorless. Their edges are generally round and they are usually slightly raised.

Hemolysis

Hemolysis is the destruction or alteration of the RBCs in the media surrounding a colony. There are two types of hemolysis:

- **Beta,** or complete, hemolysis produces a clear zone around a colony (Fig. 8-1).
- **Alpha,** or partial, hemolysis produces a greenish zone around a colony (Fig. 8-2).

The infrequently used term "gamma hemolysis" refers to nonhemolytic colonies.

1. Group A streptococci are beta hemolytic. Organisms other than streptococci can cause beta hemolysis on a sheep-blood agar plate. Be sure that any beta-hemolytic colonies selected are small and transparent. Large, opaque colonies are not likely to be streptococci.

■ **Pretest question #1:** The following statement is true. Group A streptococci produce beta hemolysis on a sheep-blood agar plate.

2. If beta-hemolytic colonies resembling streptococci are present on the plate, pick a well-isolated beta-hemolytic colony (use a sterile inoculating loop) and streak over one third to one half of the surface of a fresh sheep-blood agar plate so as to achieve a heavy, confluent growth of bacteria.
    If no beta-hemolytic colonies are seen, reincubate the plate and reexamine after an additional 24 hours incubation.
3. Place a bacitracin disk in the middle of the inoculated area and gently press the disk against the agar surface with the inoculating loop or a sterile wooden stick. Do not press the disk into the agar. It should rest just on the top of the agar.
4. Incubate the plate at 35–37°C for 18 to 24 hours.
5. After incubation, examine the area around the disk for a zone (ring) of inhibition of growth of the organism.
6. A small, transparent beta-hemolytic colony that shows any sensitivity to bacitracin is presumptively identified as a Group A streptococcus (Fig. 8-3). Note that this procedure allows **presumptive identification** of an organism as Group

(text continues on page 201)

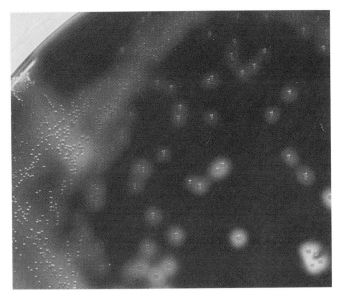

FIGURE 8-1
Beta-hemolytic colonies.

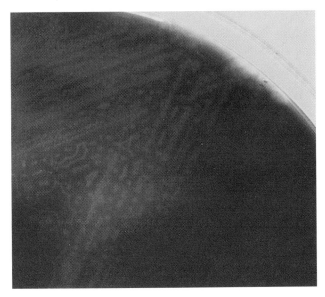

FIGURE 8-2
Alpha-hemolytic colonies.

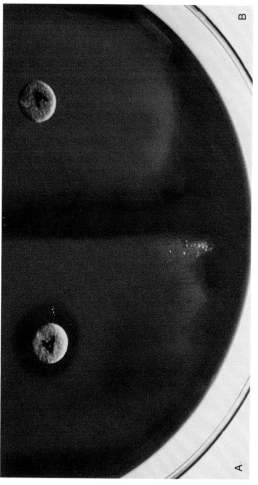

FIGURE 8-3

Beta-hemolytic sreptococci with bacitracin disk. (A) Sensitive = Group A streptococci (B) Resistant = not Group A streptococci.

A streptococcus. To identify the isolate definitively, you must do additional testing (see technical notes below). For most purposes the bacitracin disk test is adequate to diagnose streptococcal pharyngitis.

With this procedure, at least 48 hours are required for a positive result to be reported. There are procedures in use that shorten this time. Some practitioners will put a bacitracin disk on the original throat culture plate in the first area (most heavily inoculated) that is streaked with the throat culture swab. If there are many beta-hemolytic colonies on the plate, a zone of inhibition of hemolysis may be visible around the disk. However, many times there will not be a sufficient number of beta-hemolytic colonies to cause a clear zone of inhibition, and other bacteria present as normal flora in the oropharynx may be inhibited by bacitracin. For these reasons this method is not recommended.

▓▓▓ Clinical Tips

- Rare isolates of Group A streptococci will not be sensitive to bacitracin.
- Other groups of beta-hemolytic streptococci are occasionally sensitive to bacitracin.
- In order to demonstrate beta hemolysis, some isolates of Group A streptococci require an anaerobic (oxygen-free) environment.
- As an alternative to the use of bacitracin disks, commercially available latex agglutination or enzyme immunoassay tests may be used to identify Group A streptococci. The kits identify antigens (group-specific carbohydrates) on the surface of the organism and are very specific. Although these kits are more expensive, they are also more accurate in the identification of Group A streptococci.

ALTERNATIVES TO CULTURE FOR THE DIAGNOSIS OF STREPTOCOCCAL PHARYNGITIS

Many antigen detection tests (ADTs) have become available that allow the rapid identification of Group A streptococci directly from throat swabs. These tests provide rapid diagnosis (10 minutes to 2 hours) of streptococcal pharyngitis and thus facilitate the prompt initiation of appropriate antibiotic therapy. Generally, these tests are easily performed and interpreted. The specificity of these tests is quite high and therefore, a provider can treat a patient with a positive ADT without performing a throat culture.

In contrast, the sensitivity of many of these tests is significantly lower than that of a culture. An individual with a negative ADT test may still be infected with Group A streptococci. Therefore, a negative ADT should be confirmed with a throat culture, which remains the "gold standard" for diagnosis of strep throat.

■ **Pretest question #3** The following statement is true. The throat culture is the "gold standard" for the diagnosis of streptococcal pharyngitis.

If one of these kits is used, be sure to follow all manufacturers instructions for both performing the tests and doing quality control on the test reagents. Always check the expiration date of all reagents and do not use any that have expired. Most manufacturers have technical support telephone numbers to answer any questions concerning their products.

STREAKING FOR THE ISOLATION OF PURE CULTURE

To characterize and study a microorganism, it is necessary to isolate it from all other microorganisms and maintain it in pure form. This is usually accomplished by spreading a sample containing microorganisms on a solid medium so that a single cell occupies an isolated portion of the agar surface. The repeated multiplication of the single cell will eventually produce a colony that is made up of similar cells. Cultures consisting of a single species (or strain) are considered to be pure cultures.

One technique for isolating pure cultures from mixtures involves the streak-plate technique. This technique consists of spreading a small amount of culture with an inoculating loop over an agar surface. As the microorganisms are spread over the surface, single microbial cells will be deposited on an area of the agar medium, multiply, and form a colony. This colony, derived from a single cell, can then be picked with a bacteriological loop (or a needle) and subcultured onto fresh culture medium. In this way, a pure culture of an isolated colony can be obtained and maintained for study.

Quadrant Streak Method

1. Spread the organisms over a small area near the edge of the plate. This is Area 1. Apply the loop lightly to the medium to avoid digging into the agar.
2. Flame the loop and allow it to cool. Rotate the plate one third of a turn.
3. Make five or six streaks from Area 1 into Area 2. Stay near the edge of the plate as shown. Then continue streaking Area 2 without running the loop through Area 1
4. Flame the loop again and allow it to cool. Rotate the plate another one third of a turn.
5. Make five or six streaks from Area 2 into Area 3. Stay near the edge of the plate as shown. Then continue streaking Area 3 without running the loop through Area 2.
6. Flame the loop before putting it down (Fig. 8-4).

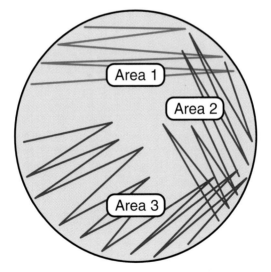

FIGURE 8-4
Streaking for isolated colonies.

CHAPTER 8 PRETEST ANSWERS

1. True. Group A streptococci produce beta hemolysis, or complete clearing, on a sheep-blood agar plate.

2. False. When doing a throat culture, the specimen swab is rolled over one third of the plate and then streaked for isolated colonies as illustrated in Figure 8-4.

3. True. Antigen detection tests are available and are very specific, but sensitivity is low. Therefore, negative antigen detection tests must be confirmed with a throat culture.

4. The tongue is depressed using a tongue blade. A sterile swab is then rolled over both tonsillar areas and lastly over the posterior pharyngeal wall. Be sure to sample any exudate that may be visible.

5. The answer is a, sheep-blood agar plate.

CHAPTER 8 POSTTEST

Question 1: Multiple choice. Select the one best answer.

1. Rheumatic fever can best be prevented by
   a. treating all carriers of Group A streptococci with penicillin.
   b. vaccination against Group A streptococci.
   c. early treatment of streptococcal pharyngitis.
   d. getting ample bed rest.

2. What is the term for partial clearing of RBCs around a colony?

3. Describe the characteristic features of *S. pyogenes* colonies on a sheep-blood agar plate.

4. Describe two methods that are used to identify an isolated bacteria as *S. pyogenes*.

5. What are the advantages and disadvantages of the ADTs that are available for the diagnosis of streptococcal pharyngitis?

CHAPTER 8 POSTTEST ANSWERS

1. The correct answer is c. In order to prevent rheumatic fever, you must adequately treat all Group A streptococcal infections.

2. Partial clearing of the RBCs around a colony is called **alpha hemolysis**.

3. *S. pyogenes* (Group A streptococci) colonies are small (<1 mm.), transparent, and surrounded by a zone of beta hemolysis.

4. a. A small, transparent colony surrounded by beta hemolysis may be **presumptively** identified as Group A streptococci by its sensitivity to bacitracin.

   b. Definitive identification requires further testing for group-specific antigens present on the organism. Commercially available kits using latex agglutination or enzyme immunoassay are available.

5. Advantages of ADTs: a. Very rapid, most kits are read after 10 minutes to 2 hours. Cultures may take 48 hours or longer for completion. b. Tests are very specific and are generally easy to interpret. Culture using bacitracin disks may give false positive results and are often difficult to interpret.

   Disadvantages of ADTs: a. Main disadvantage is that sensitivity is low and false negatives do occur. Negative ADTs should be confirmed with a bacteriological culture.

SUGGESTED READINGS

American Academy of Pediatrics. (1997). Group A streptococcal infections. In G. Peter (Ed.), *1997 Red Book: Report of the Committee on Infectious Diseases* (24th ed.), pp. 483–494. Elk Grove Village, IL: American Academy of Pediatrics.

Baron, E. J., Peterson, L. R., & Finegold, S. M. (Eds.). (1994). *Diagnostic microbiology* (9th ed.). St. Louis: Mosby.

Murphy, M. D., & Montiel, M. M. (1984). *The office laboratory in pediatrics and primary care*. Boston: G.K. Hall Medical Publishers.

Murray, P. R., Baron, E. J., Pfaller, M. A., Tenover, F. C., & Yolken, R. H. (Eds.). (1995). *Manual of clinical microbiology* (6th ed.). Washington, DC: American Society for Microbiology.

Shulman, S. T. (1994). Streptococcal pharyngitis: Diagnostic considerations. *Pediatr. Infect. Dis. J. 12,*(6), 567–570.

APPENDIX: Case Studies

Since the following case studies embrace clinical decision-making issues, the reader is encouraged to consult a primary care reference in addition to this study guide to answer the questions adequately.

CASE STUDY #1

A 30-year-old female nurse's assistant presents to the clinic with a complaint of dysuria at the beginning of micturition for the past 2 days. Associated signs and symptoms include slight vulvar burning sensation, particularly in the evening hours. She denies fever, chills, abdominal pain, back pain or any other genitourinary (G/U) signs or symptoms. Her past health history consists of a urinary tract infection (UTI) 6 months ago that was successfully treated with a 3 day course of sulfamethoxazole and trimethoprim tablets. She states that ever since she has been using the birth control pill, she has had some "vaginal itching" that occurs about once a year. She self-treats the symptom with over-the-counter miconazole cream, which consistently eliminates the symptom. Her remaining past health history is unrevealing. She has been sexually active with one male partner for the past 5 years. Her partner has no G/U complaints. She has had a pap smear and HIV antibody test 6 months ago that were both negative.

PHYSICAL EXAMINATION

Temperature: 37°C by mouth (p.o.)
    Abdomen: Nontender and without masses
    Back: Without costalvertebral angle tenderness

LABORATORY RESULTS

Midstream urinalysis: reveals macroscopic moderately (+) leuko-cyte esterase, (−) nitrite, (−) protein, (−) blood. The remaining dipstick urinalysis is unremarkable.

Figure AP-1 is a representation of 5–10 high-power fields (HPF) of the microscopic urinalysis.

QUESTIONS

1. Do the above urinalysis results adequately support a diagnosis of cystitis? State your rationale.
2. From a diagnostic perspective, what is the significance of the squamous epithelial cells in the client's midstream urine specimen?
3. Which of the following actions would you most likely do **next**? State your rationale.
   a. Treat her for cystitis.
   b. Do vaginal and pelvic examinations along with vaginal wet mounts.
   c. Send a urine specimen to the laboratory for a routine culture and susceptibility.
   d. Treat her simultaneously for a *Candida* vaginitis and lower urinary tract bacterial infection.

CASE STUDY #2

A 17-year-old high school student presents with a complaint of a small amount of white penile discharge and slight dysuria for 1 week. He has no other active health problems. He has an allergic reaction to tetracycline (a rash), and is taking no medications. He has been sexually active with the same female partner for 6 months. He has had no other sexual partners. His partner uses birth control pills. His partner has had one other male sexual partner. He states his partner is asymptomatic. He denies fever or chills; eye, ear, nose and throat signs and symptoms; rash; musculoskeletal signs and symptoms; and any other genitourinary or rectal signs.

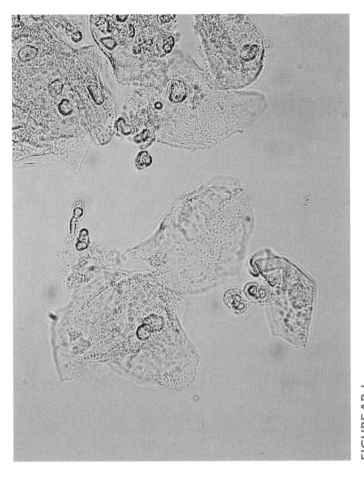

FIGURE AP-1
Microscopic urinalysis of Case Study #1.

PHYSICAL EXAMINATION

Remarkable only for a small amount of white discharge after milking his penis.

LABORATORY RESULTS

Voided urine specimen #1 (urethral specimen) is positive for 8–10 white blood cells (WBCs)/HPF, otherwise (−).

A gram stain of the urethral discharge is depicted in Figure AP-2.

QUESTIONS

1. Given the above subjective and objective data, what is the most likely diagnosis? State your rationale for your selection.
   a. Gonococcal urethritis
   b. Nongonococcal urethritis
   c. Syphilis
   d. Reiter's syndrome
2. Is it necessary to obtain urethral cultures for gonorrhea and chlamydia? State your rationale.
3. What additional diagnostic study(s) should be obtained to assess this young man's presentation? State your rationale for your selections.
   a. Saline wet mounts and KOH preparation
   b. Rapid plasma reagin (RPR)
   c. HIV antibody testing
   d. all of the above

CASE STUDY #3

A 65-year-old female who is sexually active with two male partners presents with complaints of malodorous vaginal discharge, vaginal itching, and slight dysuria for the past 3 days. Current medications include conjugated estrogen 0.625 mg qd and medroxyprogesterone acetate 2.5 mg qd. She has no other active health problems. Her past health history is negative for sexually transmitted diseases. Her partners are asymptomatic and do not consistently wear condoms. Her review of systems is otherwise noncontributory.

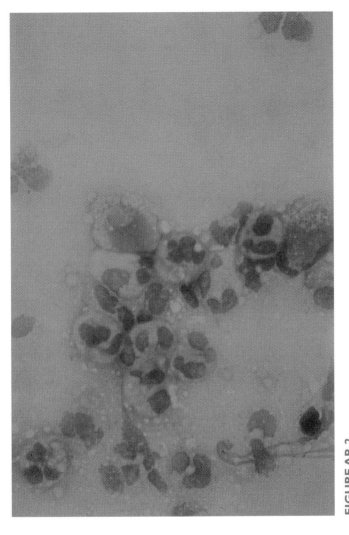

FIGURE AP-2
Gram stain of urethral discharge from Case Study #2.

PHYSICAL EXAMINATION

Temperature: 37°C p.o.

Abdomen: Nontender and without masses or hepatospleno-megaly.

Genitourinary:

External genitalia, Bartholin's glands, urethra and Skene's glands (EGBUS): erythema is noted at the introitus, no discharge, swelling or tenderness is appreciated.

Vagina: Pale pink with a moderate amount of malodorous gray-white discharge.

Cervix (Cx): Without discharge, lesions, discoloration or tenderness.

Uterus: Normal size, shape, and consistency and without tenderness or masses.

Adenexae: Nonpalpable and nontender.

Rectovaginal (RV): Without masses or tenderness.

LABORATORY RESULTS

Urinalysis with microscopic (urethral specimen and midstream): unremarkable. Saline wet mount: 20–30 WBCs/HPF otherwise (−); Potassium Hydroxide (KOH) mount- no budding yeast or psuedohyphae. Whiff test is negative.

QUESTIONS

1. What subjective and objective data from this client's presentation would support the following conditions?
   a. Trichomoniasis
   b. Bacterial vaginosis
   c. Atrophic vaginitis
2. If you suspect this woman has a *Trichomonas vaginalis* infection, why are there no motile trichomonads noted on the wet mount?
3. What are the methods for assuring visualization of trichomonads in an individual who is infected with this parasite?

CASE STUDY #4 (A, B, AND C)

Please read the following scenarios. After reading each case, determine if a fecal leukocyte test is indicated. State your rationale.

a. A mother who is breastfeeding her 2-month-old son is concerned because he has been having intermittent watery and somewhat explosive bowel movements (BMs) for the past week. The frequency of the BMs since birth has been 4 to 5 times daily. The BMs have remained a golden color, are nonodiferous and are not bloody. The baby has had no fever, nausea or vomiting. The mother has recently increased the number of fruits and vegetables in her diet as a result of having some hard BMs. The remaining history is noncontributory. The infant's temperature is 37°C via the external ear. The child has gained 1/2 kilogram since his last visit. The remaining physical examination is unremarkable.

b. A 40-year-old woman presents with a complaint of frequent (four to five), soft, brown and nonbloody BMs for the past 12 hours. Associated symptoms are slight abdominal cramping, nausea, and vomiting (two times). She thinks she may have eaten some "bad food" since a friend of hers has similar symptoms. She consults with the clinician because she thinks she may need some antibiotics. The patient appears in no apparent distress. The remaining physical examination is essentially unremarkable.

c. An 85-year-old female presents with a complaint of frequent loose BMs (five to seven per day), lower abdominal cramping, urgency, and rectal tenesmus for the past week. She is otherwise a healthy woman. Her past history is remarkable for a urinary tract infection approximately 2 weeks ago for which she was treated with amoxicillin and a sinusitis which was treated approximately 6 weeks ago with sulfamethoxazole and trimethoprim. She has had no changes in her diet and has not traveled anywhere in the past year. The remaining health history is unremarkable. The patient appears well nourished and is in no apparent distress. The patient's temperature is 37.2°C p.o.; and the blood pressure is 140/80 (lying) and 134/82 (standing). The remaining physical examination is only remarkable for some slight abdominal tenderness in the left lower quadrant of the abdomen. The fecal occult blood test is positive.

CASE STUDY #5 (A, B, AND C)

Please read the following scenarios. After reading these cases, determine which individuals should have their throats cultured for streptococcus. State your rationale.

a. A 10-year-old girl presents with a severe sore throat, tender enlarged anterior cervical lymph nodes, a temperature of 38.4°C p.o., and a frontal headache for 2 days. Her 6-year-old brother had (+) throat culture for beta-hemolytic streptococcus (Group A) and is completing a course of penicillin.

b. A 3-year-old boy is complaining of throat pain for 9 days. Associated signs and symptoms are nasal rhinitis and moist cough. He is afebrile. He is an otherwise healthy child.

c. A 50-year-old elementary school teacher is complaining of a mild sore throat and tender anterior cervical lymph nodes for 3 days. She is afebrile. She has a history of rheumatic fever at age 5. She is otherwise healthy. She takes no medications.

CASE STUDIES KEY

CASE STUDY #1

1. The clinician should have a high index of suspicion that the urinalysis results do not adequately support the diagnosis of a cystitis for the following reasons:
   a. The nitrite strip test was negative. (The nitrite test is, however, only an indirect indicator of bacteriuria. Thus, cystitis may be present despite a negative test result.)
   b. There are fewer than 10 WBCs/HPF (In a classic presentation of cystitis, there are usually more than 10 WBCs/HPF.)
   c. There are no red blood cells. (Hematuria is a common manifestation of a classic cystitis.)
   d. There are no bacteria visualized via microscopic examination. (Bacteria are often not visualized on microscopic examination of the urine, however.)
   e. Most importantly, there are numerous squamous epithelial cells noted on microscopic examination of the urine. Thus, the clinician should recognize that the urine specimen has been contaminated with urethral and/or vaginal secretions. One should then suspect that the WBCs present in the urine specimen may better reflect a diagnosis of acute urethral syndrome and/or a vaginitis rather than a diagnosis of cystitis.

2. The presence of squamous epithelial cells in a midstream urine specimen conveys to the clinician that the specimen has been contaminated with urethral and/or vulvar substances, which is usually a result of improper collection techniques.
3. The answer is "b": Do vaginal and pelvic examinations along with vaginal wet mounts.

    Since the patient is complaining of some vaginal signs and symptoms (along with the complaint of dysuria on initiation of micturition), and since the patient has a history of *Candida* vaginitis, the ambiguous urinalysis results warrant these exams and diagnostic evaluations.

Answer "a" is incorrect because there is not sufficient data to support the diagnosis of cystitis. Answer "c" should be postponed until an acute urethral syndrome and/or vaginitis have been ruled out. Answer "d" is not justified until more supporting data can be obtained (eg, findings from the vaginal and pelvic examinations and diagnostic evaluations).

CASE STUDY #2

1. The answer is "b": nongonococcal urethritis. This is the most likely diagnosis for the following reasons:
    a. The client has mild dysuria.
    b. His urethral specimen has several WBCs/HPF.
    c. There are no intracellular gram-negative diplococci seen on the Gram stain.
2. It is necessary to do urethral cultures for gonorrhea and chlamydia for the following reasons:
    a. A small subset of men with urethral exudate (~2%) who have no intracellular gram-negative diplococci on Gram stain may have a positive gonorrhea culture (Wallach, 1996). Thus, all men with a urethral exudate who have a negative Gram stain need to have a gonorrhea culture.
    b. Both cultures should be completed for individuals at high risk for sexually transmitted diseases (symptomatic and asymptomatic) given the coexistence of infection in 20%–60% of cases (Wallach, 1996).

3. The answer is "d": all of the above. In addition to gonorrhea and chlamydia, *Candida albicans* and *Trichomonas
vaginalis* may cause dysuria and urethral discharge in men.
Thus, completing a urethral wet mount (check for trichomonads) and KOH analysis (check for budding yeast
and pseudohyphae) would assist the clinician in ruling in or
out the respective infections. Note: The saline wet mount
for diagnosis of *Trichomonas* infections in men is not very
sensitive, therefore culture is recommended for diagnosis.

Since the vast majority of infectious etiologies for urethral discharge are attributable to sexual transmission, other sexually
transmitted diseases should be screened for, such as syphilis
(screening test: rapid plasma reagin) and HIV-related conditions
(screening test: HIV antibody test).

TABLE AP-1. Supportive data

Condition	Signs and symptoms	Health history	Physical examination	Diagnostics
Trichomoniasis	• Malodorous discharge • Vaginal pruritus • Dysuria	• Sexually active • Does not adhere to safe sexual practices	• Erythematous introitus • Gray-white odoriferous vaginal discharge	• Many WBCs • (−) whiff test
Bacterial vaginosis (BV)	• Malodorous discharge • Vaginal pruritus	• Sexually active (correlation with sexual transmission is unclear)	• Malodorous discharge	
Atrophic vaginitis	• Vaginal discharge may be malodorous • Vaginal pruritus • Dysuria	• Postmenopause (However, client is on hormone therapy)	• Pale vagina • Malodorous discharge	• Many WBCs

CASE STUDY #3

1. Identify subjective and objective data from this client's presentation that would support the following conditions (see Table AP-1).
2. Sensitivity of a wet mount for the detection of trichomonads is approximately 50%–70% (Wallach, 1996). An important reason for a false-negative result is a delay in the microscopic analysis of the vaginal secretions.

   Trichomonads are very temperature sensitive and will lose their mobility and die if exposed to cooler temperatures. (When trichomonads become nonmotile, it is difficult to distinguish them from WBCs.) Vaginal secretions should be examined within 15 minutes of collection to enhance the ability to detect motile trichomonads.
3. Methods for increasing the sensitivity of the vaginal wet mount would include, but are not limited to, a strict adherence to the collection and handling measures for vaginal smears as noted in Chapter 4, Diagnosis of Vaginitis/Vaginosis.

CASE STUDY #4 (A, B, AND C)

Patient a. Many clinicians would not do a fecal leukocyte examination and bacterial culture on this infant for the following reasons:

- The infant is having the same bowel pattern in terms of frequency.
- The infant is eating and sleeping well.
- The infant's watery BMs are chronologically correlated with the mother's change in dietary pattern.
- The child continues to gain weight.

Patient b. Many clinicians would defer fecal leukocyte examination and bacterial culture on this woman for the following reasons:

- The short duration of signs and symptoms
- A presentation consistent with an uncomplicated, noninflammatory diarrhea:
  - frequent loose BMs
  - vomiting
  - exposure history
  - an overall benign/nonfocal physical examination

Patient c. Fecal leukocyte examination and bacterial culture are indicated for this woman for the following reasons:

- The several-day duration of signs and symptoms
- A presentation consistent with an inflammatory diarrhea:
  - Abdominal tenderness
  - Positive fecal occult blood test
- Recent antibiotic usage (consider antibiotic-associated colitis). Toxins produced by *Clostridium difficile* cause inflammation of the intestinal mucosa and thus WBCs will be present in the fecal specimen. Routine culture for enteric pathogens will be negative. The laboratory diagnosis of *C. difficile* colitis is accomplished by detecting *C. difficile* toxins in infiltrates of stool samples.

CASE STUDY #5 (A, B, AND C)

Patient a. Many clinicians would argue that a throat culture is not necessary for this child. Since the child has enough evidence to support the diagnosis of a streptococcal pharyngitis (clinical signs and symptoms plus a solid exposure history), there is no need for this diagnostic study. Simply treat the child accordingly.

Other clinicians would argue that a throat culture is indicated because it is important to document the presence or absence of a streptococcal infection should complications ensue. The current recommendations from the American Academy of Pediatrics is to culture household contacts who have signs and symptoms suggestive of streptococcal infection.

Patient b. Most clinicians would probably not culture this child's pharynx for the following reasons:

- Child's age: Streptococcal pharyngitis is most commonly seen in children between ages 5 to 15 (Wessels, M.R. 1998).
- Child's symptom complex: In an individual who has a sore throat in conjunction with other upper respiratory signs (eg, rhinitis and cough) and is afebrile, a streptococcal pharyngitis is unlikely.

Patient c. Many clinicians would culture this woman's pharynx for the following reasons:

- Past history of rheumatic fever
- Potential exposure history given her occupation

- Presence of a sore throat without other upper respiratory signs and symptoms

REFERENCES

Bisno, A. (1991). Streptococcal infections. In Wilson, J. D. et al. (Eds.), *Harrison's principles of internal medicine*, (12th ed., pp. 563–568). New York: McGraw-Hill.

American Academy of Pediatrics. Group A streptococcal infections. In G. Peter (Ed.), (1997). *1997 Red Book: Report of the Committee on Infectious Diseases* (24th ed., pp. 483–494). Elk Grove Village, IL: American Academy of Pediatrics.

Wallach, J. (1996). *Interpretation of diagnostic tests: A synopsis of laboratory medicine*, 6th ed. Boston: Little, Brown and Company.

Wessels, M. R. (1998) Streptococcal and enterococcal infections, in Fauci, A. S. et al (eds..) *Harrison's principles of internal medicine*, (14th ed., pp. 885–892). New York: McGraw-Hill.

Lippincott Credits

Graff, L. (1983) *A handbook of routine urinalysis.* Philadelphia: J.B. Lippincott. 3–1, 3–3, 3–4, 3–5, 3–7, 3–8, 3–10, 3–11, 3–12, 3–14, 3–15, 3–16, 3–18, 3–19, 3–20, 3–21, 3–24, 3–25, 7–10B.

Garite, T. J. and Spellacy, W. N., Premature rupture of membranes (1994). N J. R. Scott et al. (Eds.) *Danforth's obstetrics and gynecology* (7th ed., pp. 305–308). Philadelphia: J.B. Lippincott. 7–7.

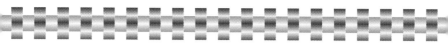

INDEX

Note: *Page numbers in* italics *indicate illustrations: those followed by t indicate tables.*